医学英语综合

高级教程

Medical English

An Advanced Integrated Course

总主编　胡继岳　杨明山

主　编　贾凌玉　沈　姝

副主编　路　璐　徐　劼

编　者　叶　玲　巩珊珊　张　燕
　　　　章国英

人民卫生出版社

图书在版编目（CIP）数据

医学英语综合高级教程 / 胡继岳，杨明山主编．—北京：人民卫生出版社，2016

ISBN 978-7-117-22102-3

Ⅰ．①医… Ⅱ．①胡… ②杨… Ⅲ．①医学－英语－医学院校－教材 Ⅳ．①R

中国版本图书馆 CIP 数据核字（2016）第 237152 号

医学英语综合高级教程

总 主 编：胡继岳　杨明山
主　　编：贾凌玉　沈　姝
出版发行：人民卫生出版社（中继线 010-59780011）
地　　址：北京市朝阳区潘家园南里 19 号
邮　　编：100021
E - mail：pmph @ pmph.com
购书热线：010-59787592　010-59787584　010-65264830
印　　刷：北京盛通印刷股份有限公司
经　　销：新华书店
开　　本：710 × 1000　1/16　　印张：17
字　　数：324 千字
版　　次：2016 年 11 月第 1 版　2016 年 11 月第 1 版第 1 次印刷
标准书号：ISBN 978-7-117-22102-3/R · 22103
定　　价：50.00 元
打击盗版举报电话：010-59787491　E-mail：WQ @ pmph.com
（凡属印装质量问题请与本社市场营销中心联系退换）

献给医学生们

献给大学英语教学改革

序

大学英语老师，事业几乎在开始的地方就可以一眼望到尽头。

英语作为大学的公共基础课程，少受重视，却也有课可上；有教材摆在面前给你教，有学生在教室等着听；上课放放PPT，有趣无趣没关系；每年两次“四”“六”级考试，怎么教成绩都差不离；这几乎成为中国高校近20年来大学英语教学的真实形态。

原以为，人生，如此而已；

原以为，可以这样一成不变地教到底……

2009年，我们发起主办了“医学人文英语论坛”——一个以学生为主体、教师为幕后、医学人文为主题、英语为工具的学生英语论坛。经过7年磨砺，论坛在国内首开先河，使得大批优秀医学生脱颖而出，他们不但能用流利的英语侃侃而谈，更是会思考、善沟通、愿奉献、能创新的复合型人才。2013年第五届医学人文英语论坛微信公众平台发布视频“小医生‘马爷’的呐喊：我们是天使还是魔鬼？”点击量超过25万人次。“医学人文英语论坛”成为全国高校英语教师们钦慕的英语教学平台，成为第二军医大学的一张靓丽的名片。

论坛让我们懂得，语言应该在使用中学习，学生的分享互动是教学最好的催化剂。

论坛让我们懂得，语言教学不必老师唱独角戏，学生才是教学的主角儿。

论坛让我们懂得，英语教材必须与学生专业紧密相关，内容和思想让英语闪亮。

2012年夏天，教研室二十多位英语老师启动了一项当时看来几乎不可能完成的任务——编写一套医学专门用途英语教材，为医科大学的学生，为大学英语改革，为这个时代，为我们自己。

讨论、争辩、调研、试讲、公开课、再讨论……循环往复，教材样章数易其稿；多少个日日夜夜，英语老师们在啃食着医学这块陌生而坚硬的骨头；为确保教材样本的科学性和客观性，老师们建立了500万词汇的医学英语语料库，生成了医学高频词汇表。2013年9月，课用教材在新生试点班开始全面试用，3年间不断修正，精益求精。

我们坚信：工作，得有意义；活着，得有趣儿。

这是一套英语老师们编写的突出听、说、读、写、译语言能力的医学英语语言类教材，既专业又通俗，既科学又人文，语言素材鲜活、原汁原味，内容广泛，以点带面，教材注重教学方法的改革，突出以学生为主体、项目为抓手的教学模式，力图打破教师一言堂，强调教师的示范、设计、指导、监管、评价等新的定位和角色，倡导注重教学过程的新型评价方法，适合医学高等院校所有专业的本科、研究生选择使用，也适合医学高等院校英语教师转型选用。

感谢第二军医大学外语教研室全体教师对本套教材的倾心付出！

感谢《生物医学研究杂志（英文版）》(*Journal of Biomedical Research*)责任主编崔波博士对本套教材的审校！

平凡如大学英语教师，也觉得这辈子应该做点什么，证明我们的存在。

这套教材，做了一个标记。

胡继岳

2016年8月

前言

上海圣约翰大学为沪上旧时之名校，莘莘学子日后成为中国各界杰出人物甚众，谓圣约翰学子影响乃至改变中国与亚洲部分现代历史绝不为过。在医学界，各科之权威来自圣约翰大学，几成当时之常态。再观崛起之亚洲邻国印度，其综合实力低中国一截，然其医疗水平却受欧美同行追捧，且其医疗管理确有过人之处。想当初，若无美国传教士卜舫济（F. L. Hawks Pott）力推英语授课之教育方式，哪有上海圣约翰这段辉煌回忆？印度若无以英语作为印度官方与教育用语，印度医生岂能执“世界医疗旅游”之牛耳！究其两者本因，莫不与语言优势相关，内外之例无不显示英语教育对于医学教育事业之巨大推力。

我国高校公共外语教学之水准已达历史最高峰。然喜中有忧，良好的公共英语基础如何有效应用于科技实践，乃是当前外语教育亟待解决的共有难题。这一“共有难题”，实为有待跨越的三个瓶颈，在医学英语教学中三类瓶颈现象尤为突出。

1. 医学英语教材的原始素材何在？

编者曾调查中国国家图书馆等五所大型图书馆馆藏医学英语类专著，检索期限自1949年至2012年，共计613种。纵观63年间的医学英语教学素材，多半源出以杂志（magazine）而非以学术期刊（academic journal）为主体的出版物。医学生与医学专业工作者同属医学专业群体，其所需主要是期刊论文而非杂志文章。若高校医学英语教学以杂志文章而非学术期刊论文作为主体教学材料，焉能要求当今医学生能够顺畅阅读学术期刊论文？此理同样适用于医学名著教学。故云原汁原味的英语医学文献和医学经典教材应该是医科大学生医学英语学习的主要素材。

2. 医学英语教材的重心何在？

原版医学文献学习，并非要求用英语教授医学，而是教授关于医学的英语语言特点和规律。例如，认知医学术语学是医学英语教学的首要教学任务。本系列中的医学英语术语教材解析医学术语学的主要规律，只要学生熟记约400个构词形，便能基本解决医学术语的认知难题。又如医学文献语法特征明显突出：①研究对象是疾病、病原及病人等，均是医学行为的承受者，故医学文献中被动语句多；②医学研究强调实验的条件与时间，故医学文献中条件状语与时间状语句多；③医学研究成果并非一蹴而就，而是从不确定状态逐渐趋于明朗，故医学文献中委婉与虚拟语句多。在此仅举数例，不一而足。

医学文献的体裁多样化也是医学英语教材无法回避的问题。不同体裁的医学文献有不同著录格式，而不同著录格式具有各自固定的句型要求，国外在医学英语写作上称 controlled language。总之，英语医学文献体裁亦是医学英语教材选材必须面对的问题，以点代面是我们的策略。

3．医学英语教学的平台何在？

医学科学研究所需信息 80% 以上来自学术期刊，而学术期刊的信息首先从医学文摘中获取。值得注意的是，印刷版的世界著名的《医学文摘索引》(*Index Medics*，*IM*) 自 2003 年起永久性停刊，被互联网上 PubMed 取而代之。随后，在《新英格兰医学期刊》等带领下，全球许多著名医学期刊陆续出版电子版。尽管供免费获取信息的是非最新期刊，但是对于以语言教学为主的医学英语教学而言，这些资源已经足够。另外，医学词典、医学动画片、医学查房、医学会议录音视频等多种医学英语教学资源在互联网上层出不穷，成为教材取之不尽的宝藏。再者，随着自媒体微信技术的普及，学生的学习成果亦可以成为分享学习的资源，教学成果既鼓励了学生，教学过程又深化了教学。教学相长真正如虎添翼，互联网在医学英语教学中的推动力和平台效应会一发而不可收。

随着上述三大瓶颈而来的，是大学公共英语教师在实际教学中所面临的两大难题，编者试图在此作出一二解答。

1．公共外语教师如何教学医学英语？

新形势下，公共外语教师不能再沿用以往“教师一言堂”的老办法来教授医学英语，而是应该创新教学模式，在陌生的医学英语教学环境下创造出新天地，走出不同的路，即 PBL（project based learning）和 SBL（students based learning）。

所谓 PBL，就医学研究生而言，是指在导师指导下，学生完成规定医学课题研究，其过程为“医学检索、文献阅读、文献翻译、文献应用、文献写作及医学交流”六个环节。医学英语学习亦然，本科生的医学英语教学也可效仿实施，只有围绕课题，结合六个研究环节，具体学习应用医学英语知识，才能切实做到学以致用。此为 PBL 教学模式，称之为基于课题或基于项目的学习。医学英语教师在教学上应贯彻“共性”原则，这是“渔”；学生的学习终端自我选择课题实施模拟 PBL，这是“鱼”。教师授之以“渔”，学生可用之于“鱼”。围绕一个课题学习终端主攻方向，教师规划、参与、监督、评估学习过程，医学英语学习可事半而功倍。PBL 是本书的学习核心模式之一，只有平时不断努力实施 PBL 模式，让医学生养成以我为主而非盲目跟从教师的学习素养，学生必然在学习过程中收获巨大。

那么，何为SBL？学习终端在工作场所，故学习者既可能是个体，也可能是集体，两者均须充分发挥学生为主导的潜在的能力，才能圆满完成学习任务。在此类医学生参与模拟的涉外门诊交流、医学查房、病例讨论、国际会议、论文答辩、实验带教等学习过程中，医学英语教师仅仅是指导者，而非学习的中心者。集体学习方式（如英语查房、模拟国际会议）可能要求学生扮演多种角色，学生既需团队协作精神，又需发挥个人才能，八仙过海各显神通。学习终端的评价可以团队成绩为基础，有别于传统的大规模选择题考试。编者相信，这样以学生为主的学习模式（SBL）让学生在模拟的实际运用中学习并演练医学英语，这种体验教学对学生熟练掌握语言并增加自信大有益处。

本系列教材的作业布置，均以上述模式作为基本理念。无论是课前、课中还是课后，教师始终是教学的指导者而非学习的中心。

2. 医学英语教师的未来何在？

医学英语脱离不了“医学”知识，故理想的医学英语教师应该是英语与医学双通的复合型人才。目前医学高校公共外语教师供大于求，而医学英语师资奇缺。要根本解决师资问题，必须依靠高校公共外语教师的自我转型，实用的实践方法就是上述的PBL，公共英语教师何不身先士卒，自我尝试一番PBL医学英语教学，闯出一条前人没有走过的路。第二军医大学的大多数青年英语教师敏而好学，敦而耐劳，边教边学，教学相长，历经数年之磨炼，磨此一剑，颇有心得，本书编撰出版是外语教研室全体教师共同努力之成果。

每逢首次医学英语授课，放映一段诺贝尔生理学或医学奖颁奖仪式，这已成为第二军医大学医学英语教学开课的一个传统。每当颁奖号声响起，教师心潮澎湃，在对国外获奖者心存崇敬的同时，难免感到一丝遗憾。终于在2015年12月11日，屠呦呦女士作为第一位获奖者，代表前赴后继的中国医学和生物学人站在了瑞典斯德哥尔摩诺贝尔奖颁奖台上，这是让国人何等骄傲和激动的时刻！

医学英语教师应勇于探索，勇于创新，为继续医学英语之中国梦而奋斗终生。

杨明山

2016年8月

Contents

Unit 1

Wonders of the Human Body

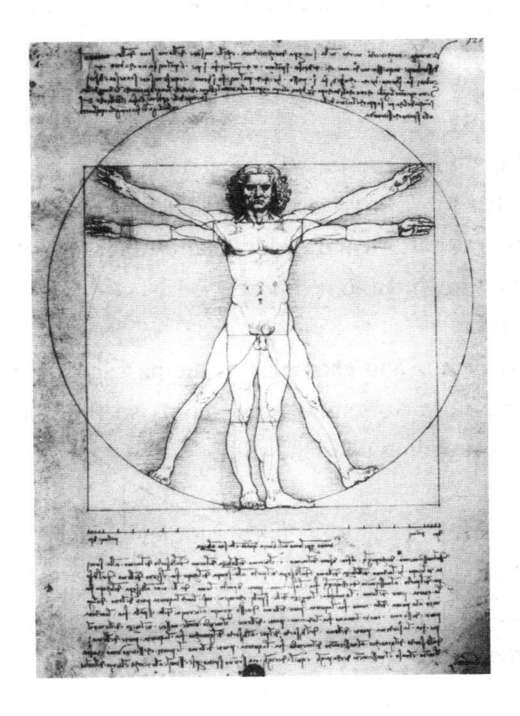

If anything is sacred, the human body is sacred.

——Walt Whitman

Skills Bank

Identifying Organizational Patterns (I)—Patterns that List

When you are trying to comprehend a passage or an essay, it is helpful to examine how the author arranges the sentences to convey his/her message. Authors want readers to comprehend the messages and ideas in a passage, so they will organize the information in a way to make it clear and easily understood. This method of organizing and arranging sentences within an essay or passage is referred to as an "organizational pattern." The most commonly used organizational patterns are patterns that list and patterns that explain and analyze.

Patterns that List

Simple listing

In this pattern, the author presents facts, details, examples, cases, ideas, and other supports in list form. It is very important to remember that in the simple listing organizational pattern the order of the items is not important for the author's meaning or argument to be understood.

Order of importance

In this pattern, the details and examples of the passage are presented in a very specific order. The author organizes the details so the most important detail comes first or last, depending upon the author's writing technique and style.

Time order

This pattern is also referred to as "chronological order." In this pattern, the author presents the events of a story or the details of a passage in the order in which they occurred in time.

Spatial/Place order

In this pattern, the author describes the location of items in relation to each other and to a larger context. In spatial/place order organizational patterns, the author creates a visual picture that permits you to "see" where various details exist in relation to other details.

Pre-class Tasks

Task 1: Medical Terminology Study

Directions: Study the word roots, prefixes and suffixes listed in the table below and do the **Vocabulary Preview** exercise for Text A or / and Text B according to your teacher's instructions.

Roots	Meaning
esophag/o	esophagus 食道
chem/o	drug; chemical 药物；化学的
my/o	muscle 肌肉
cardi/o	heart 心脏的
calci/o	calcium 钙的
coron/o	heart 心脏的
hormon/o	hormone 激素的
sebace/o	sebum 皮脂
spir/o	to breathe 呼吸
uter/o	uterus (womb) 子宫
systol/o	contraction 收缩
cyan/o	blue 青蓝
cutane/o	skin 皮肤
steth/o	chest 胸腔
fibr/o	fiber 纤维
ventricul/o	ventricle (of heart or brain) 室
Prefixes	**Meaning**
a-/an-	no; not; without 无；没有；否定
de-	lack of; removal of 缺少；去除
contra-	against; opposite 相反的
endo-	in; within 内部的
tachy-	fast 快的
Suffixes	**Meaning**
-crine	to secrete; separate 分泌；分离
-ium	structure; tissue 结构；组织
-plegia	paralysis 瘫痪；麻痹
-ia	condition 疾病
-ous	pertaining to 属于

Task 2: Prepared Individual Presentation

***Directions*:** The assigned students need to prepare a 1-min oral presentation concerning the questions in **Text-related Presentation** for Text A and / or Text B as required by your teacher.

Task 3: The Muddiest Points

Directions: Read Text A and Text B in the study group to find out the sentences that are the least clear to you after your discussions, the viewpoints that you disagree with and the understanding you have achieved through discussions and the questions you want to put forward concerning the content of the texts. Put the above information in a slip and send it to the teacher via WeChat 24 hours prior to the class. (The slip can be found on the last page of the book.)

In-class Tasks

Text A

Before You Read

Task 1: Vocabulary Preview

Directions: Divide the following words into their word parts and then give their Chinese translations by referring to **Medical Terminology Study**.

Medical Terms	Prefix	Word Root(s)	Suffix	Chinese
sebaceous				
endocrine				
esophagus				
uterus				
coronary				
asymptomatic				
ventricular				
fibrillation				
arrhythmia				
tachycardia				
cyanotic				
transcutaneous				
stethoscope				
cardioplegia				

Task 2: Warming-up

Directions: Watch the video and try to answer the questions below. While watching the video, please take notes in the blanks to help you follow the content.

1) Describe the stages of how the human body is formed.

2) What's the strongest muscle in the human body?

3) Which part of the human body is the most complex object in the world?

Notes

Text A The Human Body

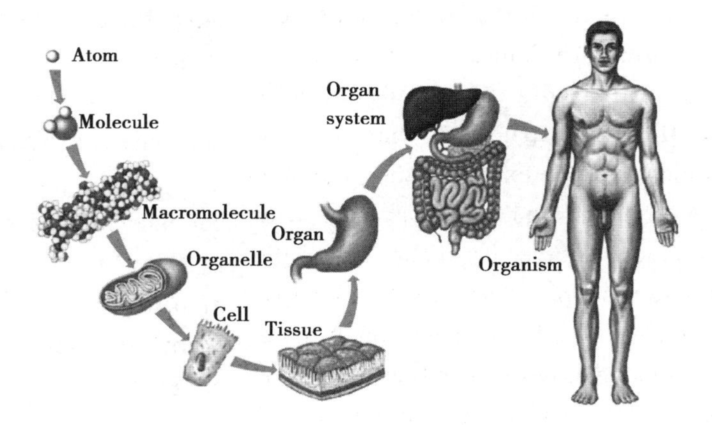

1. Anatomy is the study of the human body. It is concerned with[1] the structure of a part. For example, the stomach is a J-shaped, **pouch**-like organ. The stomach wall has thick folds, which disappear as the stomach expands to increase its capacity. Physiology is concerned with the function

pouch /paʊtʃ/ n. 袋

of a part. For example, the stomach temporarily stores food, **secretes** digestive juices, and passes on partially digested food to the small intestine. Anatomy and physiology are closely connected in that the structure of an organ suits its function. For example, the stomach's pouch-like shape and ability to expand are suitable to its function of storing food. In addition, the microscopic structure of the stomach wall is suitable to its secretion of digestive juices.

secrete /sɪ'kriːt/ v. 分泌（物质）

2. The structure of the body can be studied at different levels of organization. First, all substances, including body parts, are composed of chemicals made up of submicroscopic particles called atoms. Atoms join to form molecules, which can in turn join to form macromolecules. For example, molecules called **amino** acids join to form a macromolecule called protein, which makes up the **bulk** of our muscles. Macromolecules are found in all cells, the basic units of all living things. Within cells are **organelles**, tiny structures that perform **cellular** functions. For example, the organelle called the nucleus is especially concerned with cell reproduction; another organelle, called the **mitochondrion**, supplies the cell with energy. Tissues are the next level of organization. A tissue is composed of similar types of cells and performs a specific function. An organ is composed of several types of tissues and performs a particular function within an organ system. All of the body systems together make up the organism—such as, a human being.

amino /ə'miːnəʊ/ adj. 氨基的

bulk /bʌlk/ n. 体积，数量，容量

organelle /ˌɔːgə'nel/ n. 细胞器

cellular /'seljələ(r)/ adj. 细胞的

mitochondrion /ˌmaɪtəʊ'kɒndriən/ n. 线粒体

3. The organ systems of the body can be divided into four categories as discussed next.

Support, Movement, and Protection

4. The **integumentary** system[2] includes the skin and accessory organs, such as the hair, nails, sweat glands, and **sebaceous** glands[3]. The skin protects underlying tissues, helps regulate body temperature, contains sense organs, and even **synthesizes** certain chemicals that affect the rest of the body.

integumentary /ɪnˌtegjʊˈmentərɪ/ adj. 外皮的，包皮的

sebaceous /sɪˈbeɪʃəs/ adj. 分泌脂质的

synthesize /ˈsɪnθəsaɪz/ v. 人工合成

5. The skeletal system and the muscular system give the body support and are involved in the ability of the body and its parts to move. The skeletal system consists of the bones of the skeleton and associated **cartilage**, as well as the **ligaments** that bind these structures together. The skeleton protects body parts. For example, the skull forms a protective encasement for the brain, as does the rib cage for the heart and lungs. Some bones produce blood cells, and all bones are a storage area for calcium and **phosphorus** salts. The skeleton as a whole serves as a place of attachment for the muscles. Contraction of skeletal muscles accounts for[4] our ability to move voluntarily[5] and to respond to outside stimuli[6]. These muscles also maintain posture and are responsible for the production of body heat. Cardiac muscle and smooth muscle are called involuntary muscles because they contract automatically. Cardiac muscle makes up the heart, and smooth muscle is found within the walls of internal organs[7].

cartilage /ˈkɑːtɪlɪdʒ/ n. 软骨

ligament /ˈlɪgəmənt/ n. 韧带

phosphorus /ˈfɒsfərəs/ n. 磷

Integration and Coordination

6. The nervous system consists of the brain, spinal cord, and associated nerves. The nerves conduct nerve impulses from the sense organs to the brain

and spinal cord. They also conduct nerve impulses from the brain and spinal cord to the muscles and glands. The sense organs provide us with information about the outside environment. This information is then processed by the brain and spinal cord, and the individual responds to environmental stimuli through the muscular system.

7. The **endocrine** system consists of the hormonal glands that secrete chemicals that serve as messengers between body parts. Both the nervous and endocrine systems help maintain a relatively constant internal environment by coordinating and regulating the functions of the body's other systems. The nervous system acts quickly but has a short-lived effect; the endocrine system acts more slowly but has a more sustained effect on body parts. The endocrine system also helps maintain the proper functioning of the male and female reproductive organs.

endocrine /'endəukrain/ adj. 内分泌的

Maintenance of the Body

8. The internal environment of the body is the blood within the blood vessels and the tissue fluid that surrounds the cells. Five systems add substances to and/or remove substances from the blood: the cardiovascular, **lymphatic**, respiratory, digestive, and urinary systems.

lymphatic /lɪm'fætɪk/ adj. 淋巴的

9. The cardiovascular system consists of the heart and the blood vessels that carry blood through the body. Blood transports nutrients and oxygen to the cells, and removes waste molecules to be **excreted** from the body. Blood also contains cells produced by the lymphatic system. The lymphatic system protects the body from disease.

excrete /ɪk'skriːt/ v. 排泄或分泌

10. The respiratory system consists of the lungs and the tubes that take air to and from the lungs. The respiratory system brings oxygen into the lungs and takes carbon dioxide out of the lungs.

11. The digestive system consists of the mouth, **esophagus**, stomach, small intestine, and large intestine (colon), along with the accessory organs: teeth, tongue, salivary glands, liver, gallbladder, and pancreas. This system receives food and digests it into nutrient molecules, which can enter the cells of the body.

esophagus /ɪ'sɒfəgəs/ n. 食管

12. The urinary system contains the kidneys and the urinary bladder. This system rids the body of[8] **nitrogenous** wastes and helps regulate the fluid level and chemical content of the blood.

nitrogenous /naɪ'trɒdʒənəs/ adj. 氮的

Reproduction and Development

13. The male and female reproductive systems contain different organs. The male reproductive system consists of the testes, other glands, and various **ducts** that conduct semen to and through the penis. The female reproductive system consists of the **ovaries**, **uterine** tubes, **uterus**, vagina, and external **genitalia**. Both systems produce sex cells, but in addition, the female system receives the sex cells of the male and also nourishes and protects the **fetus** until the time of birth. (952 words)

duct /dʌkt/ n. 管
ovary /'əʊvərɪ/ n. 卵巢
uterus /'ju:tərəs/ n. 子宫
uterine /'ju:təraɪn/ adj. 子宫的
genitalia /dʒenɪ'teɪlɪə/ n. 外生殖器
fetus /'fi:təs/ n. 胚胎

Notes:

1. be concerned with: 涉及，和……有关
2. the integumentary system: 上皮组织系统
3. sebaceous glands: 皮脂腺
4. account for: 解释，说明
5. move voluntarily: 自主运动
6. respond to outside stimuli: 对外界刺激作出反应

7. the internal environment: 内环境
8. rid ...of: 解除，免除

Task: Text-related Presentation

Directions:Take turns to make a 1-min presentation on the following topics. Your presentation should be based on the text but not limited to the text. You are encouraged to present in a unique and creative way.

1) What's the relationship between anatomy and physiology? The text takes the stomach as an example to demonstrate the relationship between the two subjects. Think of another example to illustrate the question. (Para. 1)

2) Summarize the formation of the human body from atoms to organism. (Para. 2)

3) How many organ systems does the human body have? Select one of them and walk us through its structure, components and function. (Para .3-Para. 13)

After You Read

Task 1: Academic English Study

Directions: Read this section carefully and try to find more examples of formal English from Text A and Text B.

Formality

In an academic essay, you should avoid:

a. colloquial words and expressions: "stuff", "a lot of", "thing", "sort of"

b. abbreviated forms: "can't", "doesn't", "shouldn't"

c. two word verbs: "put off", "bring up"

d. sub-headings, numbering and bullet-points in formal essays - but use them in reports.

e. asking questions.

Task 2: Critical Thinking

Directions: Work in groups and discuss the following question. At the end of your discussion, each group will assign a representative to present your opinions on this issue.

There are many professions which are seemingly unrelated to anatomy but do require solid anatomical knowledge. For example, a cook needs to know the structure of a fish so as to cut the fish and cook the fish safely and effectivelly. Can you think of any other professions which may require the knowledge of anatomy?

Text B

Before You Read

Task 1: Vocabulary Preview

Directions: Preview the words in the table below and use them to describe the following pictures.

myocardium catheter radiograph porous electromagnetic transcutaneous

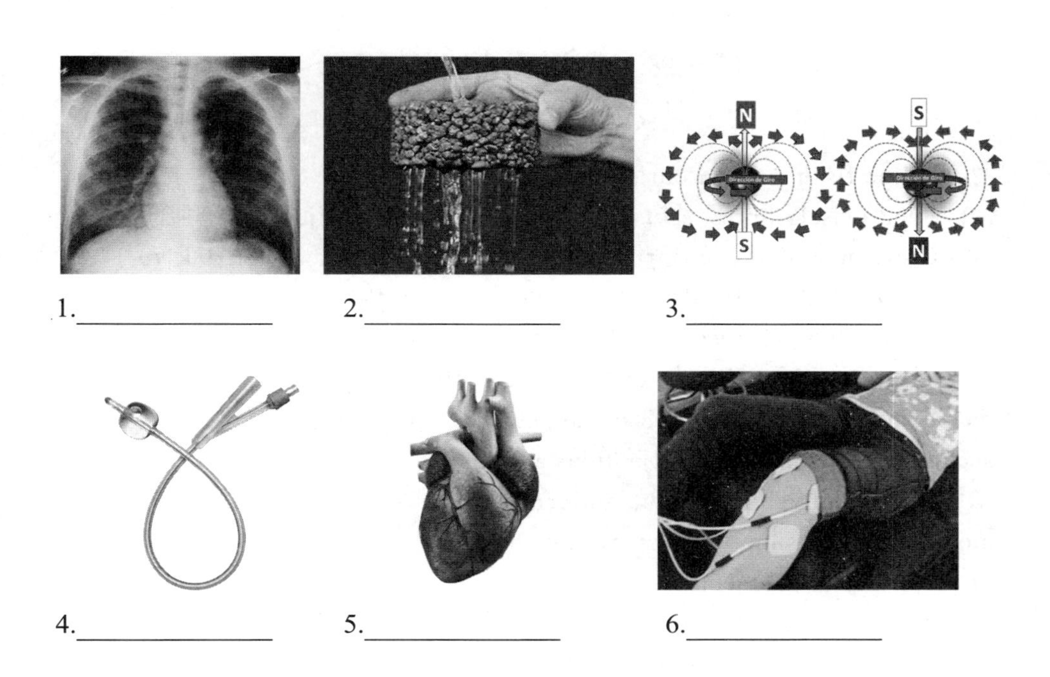

1.______________ 2.______________ 3.______________

4.______________ 5.______________ 6.______________

Task 2: Warming-up

Directions: Watch the video carefully and try to answer the questions below. While watching the video, please take notes to help you follow the content.

1) What are the functions of the heart?

2) How does it keep busy?

3) What does it look like?

Notes

Text B Unexpected Life Lessons from Cardiac Anatomy and Physiology

Sanghavi, Darshak M.

1. Cardiac tissues are a curious mixture[1] of nerve and muscle fibres, a **fusion** of electrical **conduction** and muscular release. Their surfaces contain molecular clocks that keep time by shuffling charged particles of calcium, potassium, and sodium[2] across their cell membranes. **Ion** by ion, the electrical potential[3] accumulates, as millions and billions and then trillions of ions gather. Then, suddenly, one more particle is simply too many, and a point of no return[4] is reached. The electromagnetic pressure is too great. The gates are thrown open and suddenly let the ions all crash back in, causing an electrical current to fire across the **myocardium. Systole** has begun, as the individual fibre and then the entire heart contracts.

fusion /ˈfjuːʒn/ n. 融合

conduction /kənˈdʌkʃn/ n. 传导

ion /ˈaɪən/ n. 离子

myocardium /ˌmaɪəˈkɑːdɪəm/ n. 心肌（层）

systole /ˈsɪstəli/ n. 心脏收缩

2. Like a heart, one's life requires a certain **cadence**, with alternating periods of systole and **diastole**. Sometimes I feel like one of these cardiac fibres, with periods of gathering **restlessness** followed by intense activity, and then rest again. The heart has much to teach us, by example. Muscles and people need rest between periods of intensity. Observe what happens when the example is ignored: In certain open, infected wounds, the bacterium **Clostridium** tetani[5] can grow. This organism produces a unique toxin that causes muscle cells to fire uncontrollably, in continuous systole. These contractions are called tetanic, and the name of this condition is **tetanus**. The common term "lock-jaw" refers to the uncontrolled clamping of the **masseter**, or jaw muscle. The same situation occurs in several muscles in the body, and the condition can be lethal. The lesson: diastole is critical to survival.

cadence /ˈkeɪdns/ n. 节奏
diastole/daɪˈæstəli/ n. 心脏舒张
restlessness /ˈrestləsnəs/ n. 焦躁不安
clostridium /klɒsˈtrɪdɪəm/ n. 梭菌
tetanus /ˈtetənəs/ n. 破伤风
masseter /mæˈseɪtə/ n. 咬肌

3. As a **paediatric** cardiologist, I've often reflected on the many dimensioned wisdom of the heart—not only the life lessons from the **metaphorical** emotional meanings attached to it, but those emerging from the study and appreciation of its actual physiology. Only recently, I played with a young toddler who had a **cyanotic congenital** cardiac defect with a transcutaneous oxygen saturation[6] that would have confused me. Oliver Sacks[7], the neurologist, writes that the joy of doctoring comes not from concentrating on a patient's disorder, but on his adaptation to the problem.

paediatric/ˌpiːdɪˈætrɪk/ adj. 儿科的
metaphorical /ˌmetəˈfɒrɪkl/ adj. 比喻的
cyanotic /saɪəˈnɒtɪk/ adj. 发绀的
congenital /kənˈdʒenɪtl/ adj. 先天性的

Children with heart defects have enormous physiological **resilience**. They frequently have enormous psychological resilience. Over the years, I have grown to love cardiology for this reason: it suggests to me that no problem is **insurmountable**. There in the cardiac ward, I was seeing a child do the impossible, living with an oxygen concentration previously unimaginable to me. And he was playing in front of me.

resilience /rɪ'zɪliəns/ n. 韧性

insurmountable /ˌɪnsə'maʊntəbl/ adj. 不能克服的

4. It's an unlikely teacher, this organ to which I devote my life's work. The heart is a highly disciplined structure, performing its task over and over again. The kidneys produce urine, but also regulate blood pressure, help mineralize bones, and even determine the amount of blood the bone marrow manufactures. The liver makes cholesterol, **detoxifies** wastes, and makes salts to break down fats. The pancreas regulates body sugars and makes a bevy of substances to help us digest foods. But the heart pumps blood day in and day out, without engaging in **extraneous** activities. And yet it also leaves acoustic evidence that, to the trained ear, makes every heartbeat into a diagnostic fugue[8]. A small **trill**, an extra **reverberation**, or a tiny click provides important supporting information about possible structural problems with the heart. The heart is a very public organ. Almost every event that occurs—blood entering a chamber, a heart valve opening or closing, or an extra blood vessel where it shouldn't be—leaves acoustic evidence that can be collected with a stethoscope, still another reminder that one must, first and foremost, listen to the patient.

detoxify /ˌdiː'tɒksɪfaɪ/ v. 使解毒

extraneous /ɪk'streɪniəs/ adj. 额外的

trill /trɪl/ n. 颤动声

reverberation /rɪˌvɜːbə'reɪʃn/ n. 回响

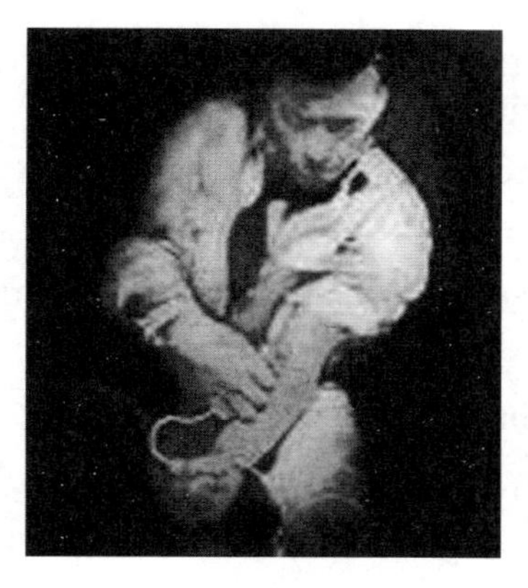

Dr. Forssmann
inserting a tube into his heart

5. Consider, also, the things people will do to learn the secrets of the heart, to unlock its meanings, to set it right. Correctly **surmising** that a tube inserted into a vein in the arm could get to the heart in 1929, the eccentric German physician Werner Forssmann[9] inserted a long **urinary catheter** deep into a vein in his own arm, until he thought it reached its destination. (A nurse had tried to stop him from performing this reckless experiment on himself, but he subdued her and tied her to an operating table.) He then walked a flight of stairs to a radiology machine, and took a **radiograph** of himself showing that the end of the catheter really had reached his heart. In this bizarre manner, Forssmann performed the world's first cardiac **catheterisation**[10], for which he later received the Nobel Prize.

surmise /sə'maɪz/ v. 猜测

urinary /'jʊərəˌneriː/ adj. 泌尿的

catheter /'kæθitə/ n. 导尿管

radiograph /'reɪdɪəʊgrɑːf / n. X线照片

catheterisation n. 导管术

6. Each minute, the heart pushes about 5 litres of blood into the **aorta**, and ultimately ejects almost 200 million litres in the typical lifetime, enough to fill a modern petroleum supertanker. And yet, at any moment for many people, the cardiac cycle goes **awry**, **deteriorating** into **fibrillation** resembling a bag of worms attempting to wriggle

aorta /eɪ'ɔːtə/ n. 主动脉

awry /ə'raɪ/ adv. 失误

deteriorate /di'tiəriəreit/ v. 恶化

fibrillation/ˌfɪbrɪ'leɪʃən/ n. 纤维性颤动

free. Roughly one in 20 adults have **asymptomatic**, short periods of **ventricular tachycardia** each day, and those with genetic defects of their potassium channels live each day **reposing** under their own sword of Damocles[11], always aware of the **transience** of their existence. Some live their lives in fear, as various subtypes of their disorders allow the most benign daily experiences-the buzz of an alarm clock, the sudden touch of water in a swimming pool—to **precipitate** lethal **arrhythmias**, from which only a precisely delivered shock can jolt them back into the world of the living. From this horrible existence, perhaps there is a reminder, as Henry David Thoreau[12] might ask, for us to constantly ask whether we are truly living sincerely, as if every day could be our last.

asymptomatic /ˌeɪsɪmptəˈmætɪk/ adj. 无临床症状的
ventricular /venˈtrɪkjʊlə/ adj. 心室的
tachycardia n. 心动过速
repose /rɪˈpəʊz/ v. 休息
transience /ˈtrænzɪəns/ n. 短暂
precipitate /prɪˈsɪpɪteɪt/ v. 突然引发
arrhythmia /əˈrɪθmɪə/ n. 心律失常

7. Centuries ago, blood was thought to have sloshed in a disorderly manner throughout the body, and the heart considered a porous organ of no clear mechanical significance. William Harvey[13], a 17th-century Oxford physician, examined the blood vessels of almost 80 different animals, including dogs, fish, and man, and discovered an unusual property of veins. When he forced water through veins towards the heart, the water passed without resistance. However, when he tried to inject water in the opposite direction, it would not pass. Harvey realized that blood circulates in a single direction, and that the heart is a mechanical pump.

8. Periodically, I observe the opening of a person's chest during cardiac surgery, and it is always a magnificent and terrible sight. Not so long ago, I watched a young, brain dead teenage boy whose heart continued beating, **oblivious** to[14] the absence of its master. Slightly larger than a softball, the adolescent's heart alternately swelled and collapsed in an orderly top to bottom fashion, about once every second. It had done this without pause for the past 17 years, hidden until today. Soon, the surgeons infused the ice-cold **cardioplegia** solution[15] and the heart collapsed within the chest.

oblivious /əˈblɪviəs/ adj. 未察觉的

cardioplegia /kɑːdiəuˈpliːdʒiə/ n. 心麻痹

9. His heart stopped when there was no longer any reason to pump, no longer any life-blood to circulate. A heart can't beat, it seemed, without something nourishing to fill it. I thought again about Harvey, who in some sense stripped the heart of its metaphors when he found it was only a pump. Yes, I thought with a sense of loss, looking at the limp muscle that beat moments ago. It was just a pump. And yet, this pump was enough for the child who would soon accept the donated organ. And it would always carry this **fervent** message from the parents who **relinquished** it: please take this gift, so **suffused** with our hopes and dreams and yet, in the end, simply a cord of muscle that we hope will beat for decades to come, sustaining the life of the one you love and transcending the body of the one whom we loved. (1277 words)

fervent /ˈfɜːvənt/ adj. 热烈的

relinquish /rɪˈlɪŋkwɪʃ/ v. 放弃（要求等）

suffuse /səˈfjuːz/ v. 弥漫于某物，布满

Notes:

1. curious mixture: 奇妙的组合

2. charged particles of calcium, potassium, and sodium: 带电的钙钾钠离子
3. electrical potential: 电势，电位
4. a point of no return: 极限点，不能回头的地步
5. clostridium tetani: 破伤风杆菌，破伤风梭状芽胞杆菌，破伤风芽孢梭菌
6. cyanotic congenital cardiac defect with a transcutaneous oxygen saturation: 指的是紫绀性先天性心脏缺陷，发病原因是经皮血氧饱和度低，导致颜面、口唇青紫（发绀）。
7. Oliver Sacks: 人名，神经病学专家，在医学和文学领域均享有盛誉。被书评家誉为20世纪难得一见的“神经文学家”。
8. diagnostic fugue: 诊断的赋格曲。在音乐术语中，赋格曲指的是一种特殊的音乐形式，它以简单的音调开始，然后将同一音调用不同的乐器或声调加以演奏。此处将心脏正常的声音夹杂着变化后的声音比作赋格曲，通过聆听这种变化的声音可以诊断出心脏的疾病。
9. Werner Forssmann: 人名，德国外科医生。因发明心脏导管术而获得1956年诺贝尔生理学或医学奖。
10. cardiac catheterization: 心脏导管术
11. sword of Damocles: 达摩克利斯之剑，中文或称“悬顶之剑”，用来表示时刻存在的危险。源自古希腊传说：迪奥尼修斯国王请他的大臣达摩克利斯赴宴，命其坐在用一根马鬃悬挂的一把寒光闪闪的利剑下，由此而产生了这个外国典故，意指令人处于一种危机状态，“临绝地而不衰”。或者随时有危机意识，心中敲起警钟等。
12. Henry Da Thoreau: 人名，美国作家，诗人，哲学家，历史学家，代表作有《瓦尔登湖》(*Walden*)。
13. William Harvey: 人名，英国17世纪著名的生理学家和医生。他发现了血液循环的规律，奠定了近代生理科学发展的基础。
14. oblivious to: 形容词短语，意为对……没有察觉到。
15. cardioplegia solution: 心脏停搏液，使心脏达到电机械停搏状态。

While You Read

Task 1: Reading Skills Practice

Directions: Read text B carefully and try to identify the organizational patterns in this article. Find in the corresponding paragraphs detailed information about the methods used. (See ***Skills Bank***)

Organizational patterns	Methods	Detailed information	Para.
Simple listing	facts		
	details		
	examples		
	cases		
	ideas		
	others		

Task 2: Text-related Presentation

Directions:Take turns to make a 1-min presentation on the following topics. Your presentation should be based on the text but not limited to the text. You are encouraged to present in a unique and creative way.

1) Explain the systole and diastole of the heart. (Try to introduce the mechanism in a vivid and easy-to-understand way) (Para.1)

2) Explain the term "clostridium tetanus". (Para.2)

3) Give a brief introduction of cyanotic congenital cardiac defect. (Para. 3)

4) What's physiological and psychological resilience? What characteristics do resilient people have in common? (Para.4)

5) Tell us how Werner Forssmann discovered catheterization surgery (You can also add the modern application of catheterization and his secrets of success)(Para.5)

6) Give us a brief introduction of Harvey and his blood circulation theory (If possible, present the special qualities that lead him to the great discovery) (Para.8)

After You Read

Task 1: Oral Presenting

Directions: Try to rephrase or explain the following sentences without using the boldfaced words or phrases. (This is going to be integrated into the communicative interaction in the classroom. The task can be done orally in the classroom.)

1. Over the years, I **have grown to love** cardiology for this reason: **it suggests to me** that no problem is **insurmountable**. There in the cardiac ward, I was seeing a child do the impossible, living with an oxygen concentration previously **unimaginable to me**. And he was playing in front of me.
2. As a paediatric cardiologist, I've often **reflected on** the many dimensioned wisdom of the heart-not only the life lessons from the metaphorical emotional

meanings **attached to** it, but those emerging from the study and **appreciation** of its actual physiology.

3. Oliver Sacks, the neurologist, writes that the **joy of doctoring** comes not from **concentrating on** a patient's disorder, but on his **adaptation to** the problem.
4. Some live their lives in fear, as various subtypes of their disorders allow the most benign daily experiences-the buzz of an alarm clock, the sudden touch of water in a swimming pool—to **precipitate lethal arrhythmias**, from which only a **precisely delivered shock** can **jolt them back** into the world of the living.
5. Please take this gift, so **suffused with** our hopes and dreams and yet, in the end, simply a cord of muscle that we hope will beat for decades to come, **sustaining the life** of the one you love and **transcending** the body of the one whom we loved.

Task 2: Critical Thinking

Directions: Work in groups and discuss the following question. At the end of your discussion, each group will make a list of your key points and select a reporter to present your opinions. The group members should take turns to report and take notes in this semester.

A saying goes that people fail for the same reason yet the secrets for their success may vary. Please discuss the example of Harvey and Forssmann, two of the greatest medical pioneers mentioned in Text B and try to sum up the reasons for their success. If possible, can you support your opinions with the examples of some other successful people?

After-class Tasks

Task 1: Word Chunks

Directions: Complete the following word chunks taken from Text A and Text B according to their Chinese equivalents and make a sentence with each word chunk.

1. ________ organs 内脏
2. ________ temperature 调节体温
3. ________ glands 内分泌腺
4. nerve ________ 神经冲动
5. ________ digestive juice 分泌消化液
6. the ________ system 骨骼肌肉系统
7. the ________ system 生殖系统
8. ________ cardiac defect 先天性心脏缺陷
9. physiological ________ 心理韧性
10. ________ chemicals 合成化合物
11. ________ organ 高度自律的器官
12. ________ fats 分解脂肪
13. a ________ experiment 鲁莽的实验
14. ________ food 储存食物
15. the ________ system 上皮组织系统
16. ________ the life 维持生命
17. ________ rate 死亡率
18. the ________ system 消化系统
19. the ________ system 神经系统
20. the ________ system 心血管系统

Task 2: Translation

Directions: Translate sentence 1 to 3 into Chinese and pay close attention to the translation of the words in bold. Then translate sentence 4 to 6 into English using the words in the bracket.

1. Contraction of skeletal muscles **accounts for** our ability to move voluntarily and to respond to outside stimuli.

____

____

2. The surface was largely covered by **glistening** yellow fat, its normal coat. A few worm-like structures were also **visible** below that fat; these were the coronary arteries, the blood vessels that give oxygen to the heart.

____

____

3. Not so long ago, I watched a young, brain dead teenage boy whose heart continued beating, **oblivious to the absence of** its master.

____

____

4. 一个刚蹒跚学步的孩子患有因经皮血氧饱和度低而导致的紫绀性先天性心脏缺陷。(congenital, cyanotic)

____

____

5. 肾脏生成尿液，控制血压，决定骨髓造血量；肝脏合成胆固醇以解毒代谢废物，分泌胆盐来分解脂肪；胰腺控制血糖，产生大量物质帮助食物消化。(detoxify, break down)

____

____

6. 每二十个成人中就有一个每天会出现短时性室性心动过速，并无明显症状。(asymptomatic)

____

____

Task 3: Listening & Speaking

Directions: Watch the video *Wonders of the Human Body* and take down notes under the three clues listed below.

1) The principles underlying the brain surgery.

____

____

2) The location of the brain and the function of each location.

Location:

____

____

Function:

____

____

3) Gifts of Van Gogh

____

Task 4: Research

Directions: Do some research into the ***history of anatomy introduce the major development of anatomy including the significant events and people and analyze the reasons for its deve lopment.*** You can present in the form of an interview, short play or simply a lecture. Make sure each member of the group will present his or her part on the stage.

Resources

Here are some websites where you can find useful information for your research.

http://www.historyworld.net/wrldhis/PlainTextHistories.asp?historyid=aa05

http://www.metmuseum.org/toah/hd/anat/hd_anat.htm

http://www.nlm.nih.gov/exhibition/dreamanatomy/da_timeline_anatomy.html

Task 5: Writing

Directions: Anatomy class must be both challenging and rewarding to any medical student. Has your anatomy class ever provoked your thoughts or touched your heart? Write an essay titled ***Reflections on My Anatomy Class***.

Task 6: Vocabulary Log

Directions: Please finish the vocabulary log (Please find the log at the end of the book) by looking up the dictionary and write down the words or expressions you have learnt in this unit by following the examples already listed in the log. And then write down the translation for each vocabulary item and if possible, its variants, synonym, antonym and the frequent collocations.

Task 7: Reading Log

Directions: After learning the whole unit and conducting the research, you have known more about human body from different perspectives. You can go to the library or surf on the internet for more knowledge about it. You can take down the key information according to the sample chart. (Please find the chart at the end of the book) Also you are allowed to complete the chart on a computer or tablet so that this section is expandable if you want to write more than the space on a paper form might allow. And then send it to your teacher by emails. The reading log can serve as an informal way to keep track of your reading progress.

Unit 2

Secrets of Cells

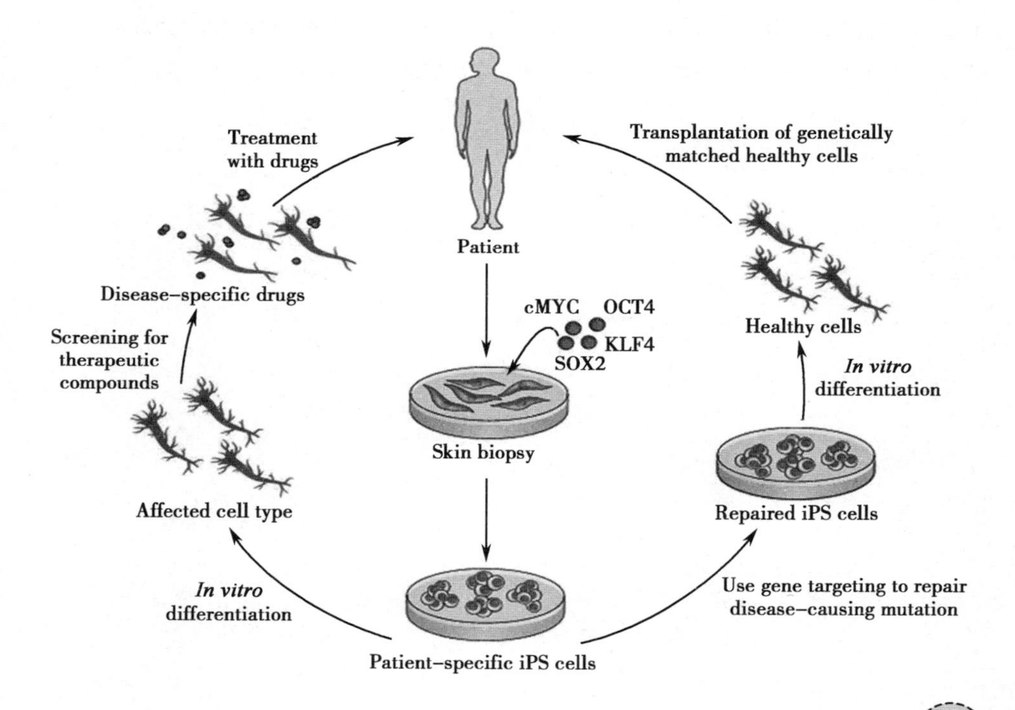

We are made of cells. And of stars. The Universe outside of us has made the universe inside us.

——L.L. Larison Cudmore

Skills Bank

Identifying Organizational Patterns (II) ——Patterns that Explain and Analyze

Example/Illustration

This pattern is also known as "generalization and example." In this pattern a general statement is made and then supported with multiple examples, with specific cases, or with an extended illustration. When an author illustrates a point, he/she shows you the point by providing specific examples and details.

Clarification

This organizational pattern is also known as "statement and clarification" or "generalization and clarification". In this organizational pattern the author uses repetition to simplify or more fully explain certain terms, ideas, or concepts. The clarification organizational pattern attempts to clarify the author's point by examining its meaning two, three, four, or more times.

Definition

In this organizational pattern, the author attempts to clarify a term or phrase with a brief or an extended definition. More than one type of definition may be used in this organizational pattern. The author may use a standard dictionary-style definition (denotation) or he/she may focus on the word's connotation. Denotation refers to the literal meaning of a word, while connotation refers to the shades of meaning associated with a word. The author's task when using the definition organizational pattern is to focus on the features that make the term or concept distinctly apart from other similar terms and concepts.

Division/Classification

In the division organizational pattern, the author takes apart a whole by dividing it into sections for further explanation. Division is similar to analysis, since the author is breaking down a larger entity to examine the component parts.

In the classification organizational pattern, the author takes the division organizational pattern one step further. In the classification organizational pattern the individual sections and categories that share characteristics with other concepts or subjects are presented.

Cause/Effect

In the cause/effect organizational pattern the author explains why or how things happen and what the result of these actions may be or might be. The cause is the source of a certain outcome. The cause is the reason or the motive behind the results. The effect is this outcome or result. The effect is the consequence of the cause that preceded it.

Compare/Contrast

To clarify, it is important to note that the compare and the contrast organizational patterns are often joined together. When an author weighs alternatives, or takes two choices, objects, or ideas and considers their similarities and differences, the organizational pattern is compare/contrast.

Pre-class Tasks

Task 1: Medical Terminology Study

Directions: Study the word roots, prefixes and suffixes listed in the table below and do the **Vocabulary Preview** exercise for Text A or / and Text B according to your teacher's instructions.

Roots	Meaning
embry/o	embryo 胚胎
nucle/o	nucleus 原子核
insulin/o	insulin (pancreatic hormone) 胰岛素
vagin/o	vagina 阴道
reticul/o	network 网络
coll/a	glue 胶
home/o	sameness; unchanging; constant 相同；不变；恒定
tub/o	tube 管道
epitheli/o	skin; epithelium 上皮
ovul/o	egg 卵子
spher/o	globe-shaped 球形
Prefixes	**Meaning**
ultra-	beyond; excess 超出；过多
retro-	behind; back; backward 逆向
dia-	complete; through 全部；相通

续表

Suffixes	Meaning
-fication	process of making 过程
-ar	pertaining to 属于……的
-blast	embryonic; immature cell 胚胎的；未成熟细胞

Task 2: Prepared Individual Presentation

Directions: The assigned students need to prepare a 1-min oral presentation concerning the questions in **Text-related Presentation** for Text A and/or Text B as required by your teacher.

Task 3: The Muddiest Points

Directions: Read Text A and Text B in the study group to find out the sentences that are the least clear to you after your discussions, the viewpoints that you disagree with and the understanding you have achieved through discussions and the questions you want to put forward concerning the content of the texts. Put the above information in a slip and send it to the teacher via WeChat 24 hours prior to the class. (The slip can be found on the last page of the book.)

Text A

Before You Read

Task 1: Vocabulary Preview

Directions: Divide the following words into their word parts and then give their Chinese translations by referring to **Medical Terminology Study**.

Medical Terms	Prefix	Word Root(s)	Suffix	Chinese
ovum				
spherical				
epithelial				
retrovirus				
tubular				
homogenous				

续表

Medical Terms	Prefix	Word Root(s)	Suffix	Chinese
invagination				
collagen				
reticular				
embryologist				
ultraviolet				
fibroblast				

Task 2: Warming-up

Directions: Watch the video carefully and try to answer the questions below. While watching the video, please take some notes in the blanks to help you to memorize the information.

1) How important are cells to our body?

2) How do cells repair our body in case of mishaps?

3) How do cells work together in the heart?

Notes

Text A A Society of Cells

1. The simplest structural units into which a complex **multicellular** organism can be divided and still **retain** the functions characteristic of life are called cells. One of the unifying **generalizations** of biology is that

multicellular /mʌltɪ'seljʊlə/ adj. 多细胞的

retain /rɪ'teɪn/ v. 保住

certain fundamental activities are common to almost all cells and represent the **minimal** requirements for maintaining cell integrity and life. Thus, a human liver cell and an **amoeba** are remarkably similar in their means of exchanging materials with their immediate environments, of obtaining energy from organic nutrients, of synthesizing complex molecules, and of **duplicating** themselves.

2. Each human organism begins as a single cell, the **fertilized ovum**, which divides to form two cells, each of which divides in turn, resulting in four cells, and so on. If cell **multiplication** were the only event occurring, the end result would be a **spherical** mass of identical cells. During development, however, each cell becomes specialized in the performance of a particular function, such as developing force and movement (muscle cells) or generating electric signals (nerve cells). The process of transforming an unspecialized cell into a specialized cell is known as cell **differentiation**. In addition to differentiating, cells **migrate** to new locations during development and form selective **adhesions** with other cells to form multicellular structures. In this manner, the cells of the body are arranged in various combinations to form a **hierarchy** of organized structures. Differentiated cells with similar properties **aggregate** to form tissues (nerve tissue, muscle tissue, and so on), which are linked together to form organ systems.

generalization /ˌdʒenərəlaiˈzeiʃən/ n. 概论，泛化

minimal /ˈmɪnɪməl/ adj. 最低的

amoeba /əˈmiːbə/ n. 变形虫

duplicate /ˈdjuːplɪkeɪt/ v. 复制

fertilize /ˈfɜːtəlaɪz/ v. 使受精

ovum /ˈəʊvəm/ n. 卵细胞

multiplication /ˌmʌltɪplɪˈkeɪʃn/ n. 增殖

spherical /ˈsferɪkl/ adj. 球形的

differentiation /ˌdɪfəˌrenʃɪˈeɪʃn/ n. 分化

migrate /maɪˈgreɪt/ v. 迁徙

adhesion /ədˈhiːʒn/ n. 粘连的组织

hierarchy /ˈhaɪərɑːkɪ/ n. 等级制度

aggregate /ˈægrɪgət/ v.（使）聚集

3. About 200 distinct kinds of cells can be identified in the body in terms of differences in structure and function. When cells are classified according to the broad types of function they perform, however, four categories emerge: (1) muscle cells, (2) nerve cells, (3) **epithelial** cells, and (4) connective-tissue cells. In each of these functional categories, there are several cell types that perform variations of the specialized function. For example, there are three types of muscle cells-**skeletal**, **cardiac**, and smooth-muscle cells—all of which generate forces and produce movement but differ from each other in shape, in the mechanism controlling their **contractile** activity, and in their location in the various organs of the body.

epithelial /ˌepɪ'θiːlɪəl/ adj. 上皮的

skeletal /'skelətl/ adj. 骨骼的

cardiac /'kɑːdiæk/ adj. 心脏的

contractile /kən'træktaɪl/ adj. 有收缩性的

4. Muscle cells are specialized to generate the mechanical forces that produce force and movement. They may be attached to bones and produce movements of the **limbs** or **trunk**. They may be attached to skin, as for example, the muscles producing facial expressions, or they may enclose hollow **cavities** so that their **contraction expels** the contents of the cavity, as in the case of the pumping of the heart. Muscle cells also surround many of the tubes in the body—blood vessels, for example—and their contraction changes the **diameter** of these tubes.

limb /lɪm/ n. 四肢

trunk /trʌŋk/ n. 躯干

cavity /'kævəti/ n. 腔

contraction /kən'trækʃn/ n. 收缩

expel /ɪk'spel/ v. 驱除

diameter /daɪ'æmɪtə(r)/ n. 直径

5. Nerve cells are specialized to **initiate** and **conduct** electric signals, often over long distances. The signal may influence the initiation of new electric signals in other nerve

initiate /ɪ'nɪʃieɪt/ v. 发起

conduct /kən'dʌkt/ v. 传导

cells, or it may influence **secretion** by a gland cell or contraction of a muscle cell. Thus, nerve cells provide a major means of controlling the activities of other cells. Their activity also **underlies** such phenomena as consciousness, **perception** and **cognition**.

6. Epithelial cells are specialized for the selective secretion and absorption of ions and organic molecules. They are located mainly at the surfaces that either cover the body or individual organs or else line the walls of various **tubular** and hollow structures within the body. Epithelial cells, which rest on a **homogenous** noncellular material called the basement **membrane**, form the boundaries between **compartments** and function as selective barriers regulating the exchange of molecules across them. For example, the epithelial cells at the surface of the skin form a barrier that prevents most substances in the external environment from entering the body through the skin. Epithelial cells are also found in glands that form the **invagination** of the epithelial surfaces.

7. Connective-tissue cells, as their name implies, have as their major function connecting, **anchoring**, and supporting the structures of the body. These cells typically have a large amount of **extracellular** material between them. The cells themselves include those in the loose **meshwork** of cells and

secretion /sɪˈkriːʃn/ n. 分泌

underlie /ˌʌndəˈlaɪ/ v. 说明

perception /pəˈsepʃn/ n. 知觉

cognition /kɒgˈnɪʃn/ n. 认知

tubular /ˈtjuːbjələ(r)/ adj. 管状的

homogenous /həˈmɒdʒənəs/ adj. 同质的，同源的

membrane /ˈmembreɪn/ n. 膜

compartment /kəmˈpɑːtmənt/ n. 分隔间

invagination /ɪnˌvædʒɪˈneɪʃən/ n. 内陷

anchor /ˈæŋkə(r)/ v. 固定

extracellular/ˌekstrəˈseljʊlə/ adj. 细胞外的

meshwork /meʃˌwɜːk/ n. 网状物

fibers underlying most epithelial layers plus other types as diverse as fat-storing cells, bone cells, and red and white blood cells. Many connective-tissue cells secrete into the fluid surrounding them molecules that form a **matrix** consisting of various types of protein fibers **embedded** in a ground substance made of complex sugars, protein, and **crystallized** minerals. This matrix may vary in consistency from a **semifluid** gel, in loose connective tissue, to the solid crystallized structure of bone. These extracellular fibers include ropelike **collagen** fibers, which have a high **tensile** strength and resist stretching, rubber-band-like **elastin** fibers, and fine, highly branched **reticular** fibers. (790 words)

matrix /ˈmeɪtrɪks/ n. 基质
embed /ɪmˈbed/ v. 嵌入
crystallize /ˈkrɪstəlaɪz/ v. 使结晶
semifluid /ˈsemɪˈfluːɪd/ adj. 半流质的
collagen /ˈkɒlədʒən/ n. 胶原蛋白
tensile /ˈtensəl/ adj. 拉力的
elastin /ɪˈlæstɪn/ n. 弹性蛋白
reticular /rɪˈtɪkjʊlə/ adj. 网状的

While You Read

Task 1: Text-related Presentation

Directions: Take turns to make a 1-min presentation about the following topics. Your presentation should be based on the text but not limited to the text. You are encouraged to present in a unique and creative way.

1) Explain “maintaining cell integrity and life”. You can refer to the example in the text or you can come up with other examples to demonstrate your understanding. (Para.1)

2) Show the process of cell differentiation with pictures. (Para.2)

3) Among the four broad categories of cells, several cell types perform variations of the specialized function. Give more examples. (Para.3)

4) Choose one cell type from muscle cell, nerve cell, epithelial cell and connective-tissue cell and elaborate on its role in the human body.

After You Read

Task 1: Academic English Study

Directions: Read this section carefully and find more examples as shown below from Text A and Text B.

Accuracy

In academic writing you need to be accurate in your use of vocabulary. Do not confuse, for example, "phonetics" and "phonology" or "grammar" with "syntax". Choose the correct word from, for example, "meeting", "assembly", "gathering" or "conference".

Or from: "money", "cash", "currency", "capital" or "funds".

You also need to be accurate in your use of grammar.

Task 2: Critical Thinking

Directions: Work in groups and discuss the following question. At the end of your discussion, each group will assign a representative to present your opinions on this issue.

Think of a good metaphor for the cell that helps us understand the organelles, their functions and how they work together. An example would be: A cell is a school with all of the organelles in the cell working together like the elements of the school do, so it can run smoothly.

Text B

Before You Read

Task 1: Vocabulary Preview

Directions: Preview the words in the table below and use them to describe the following pictures.

embryo	neuron	skeleton
cloning	genome	transplantation

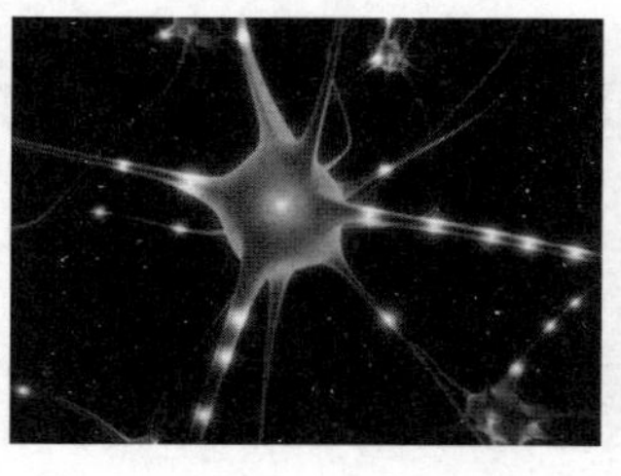

1.______________

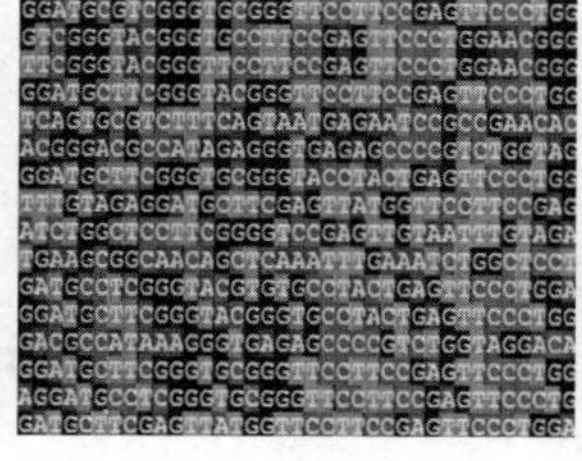

2. ______________

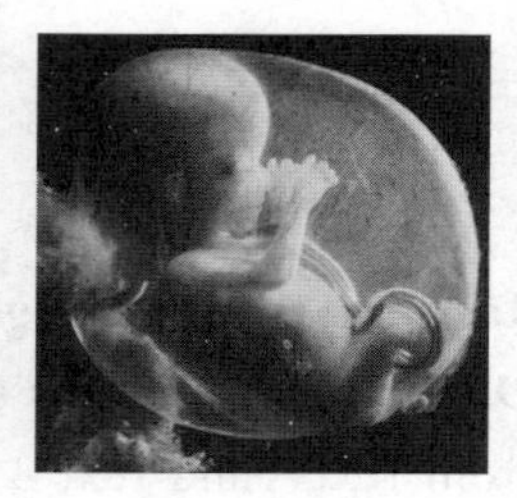

3.______________

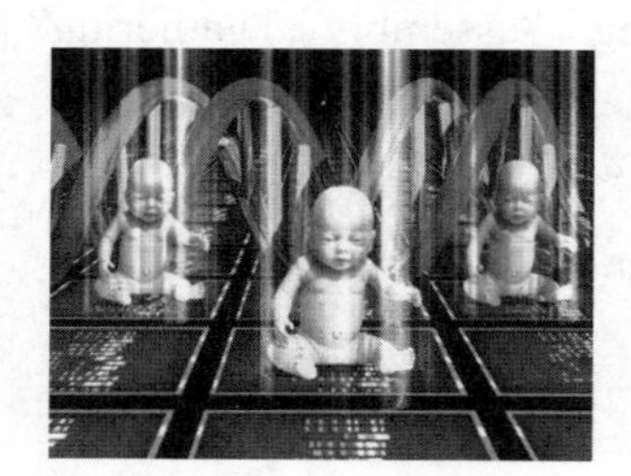

4. ______________

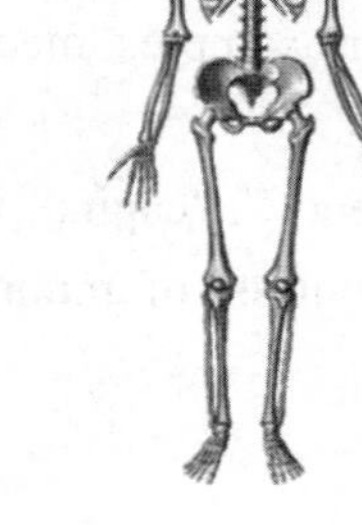

5. ______________

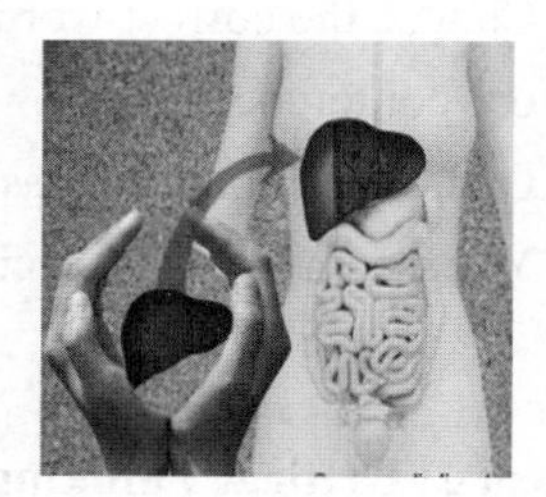

6. ______________

Task 2: Warming-up

Directions: Watch the video carefully and try to answer the questions below. While watching the video, please take some notes in the blanks to help you to memorize the information.

(1) What are stem cells? How many types of stem cells are there and what are they?

(2) What are some of the medical applications of stem cells?

Notes

Text B The Nobel Prize in Physiology or Medicine 2012

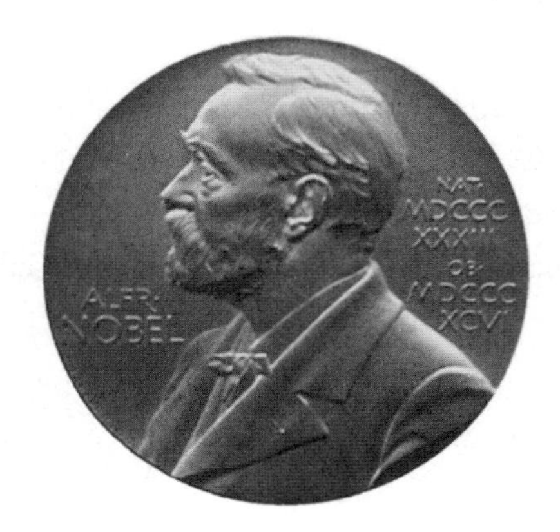

A one-way journey?

1. What are you going to be when you grow up? When you are a child, all life's paths lie open and the question has no answer. But as you move through life a long series of choices and external factors **nudge** you in a certain direction. When you grow up, maybe you will realize your inner potential by becoming a researcher or a journalist or a politician -- but probably not all at the same time.

nudge /nʌdʒ/ v. 推动

2. The cells in our body follow a similar life course. Each individual stem cell in the early **embryo** could potentially develop into any of the various types of cells that make up the adult body. These **versatile** cells are called **pluripotent** stem cells. Soon they start to develop along different pathways to take on specific tasks in the body. Some will become neurons, long thin cells that specialize in sending and receiving nerve impulses; others

embryo /'embriəʊ/ n. 胚胎

versatile /vəːsətail/ adj. 多功能的

pluripotent /plʊə'rɪpətənt/ adj. 多能的

will turn into the muscle cells that allow us to move, or the bone cells that make up our skeleton.

3. For a long time, researchers believed that life's one-way journey also applied to cells. The **doctrine** was that once a cell had developed into a specialized cell—a cell with a specific task to do in the body—it had **irretrievably** lost all the alternative possibilities that had been open to it in the beginning.

doctrine /ˈdɒktrɪn/ n. 学说

irretrievably /ˌɪrɪˈtriːvəblɪ/ adv. 不可挽回地

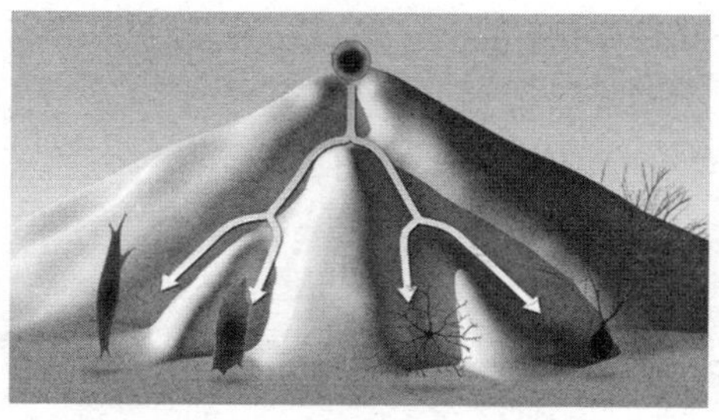

A frog-hop backwards in development

4. But in 1962 the young **embryologist** John B. Gurdon[1] presented new research findings that ran counter to the theory of life's one-way street. Not many believed him at first, but the fact remains: in his laboratory in Oxford, cell **nuclei**, containing the cell's genetic material, had jumped backwards in their development.

embryologist /ˌembrɪˈɒlədʒɪst/ n. 胚胎学家

nucleus /ˈnjuːklɪəs/ n. 细胞核（其复数形式为 nuclei）

5. John B. Gurdon suspected that every cell in the body still contained all the genetic information needed to produce all the body's various cell types, and he used an **ingenious** method to test his **hypothesis**. In his experiments, he first emptied a frog's egg of its genetic material by destroying the egg

ingenious/ɪnˈdʒiːniəs/ adj. 巧妙的，灵巧的

hypothesis /haɪˈpɒθəsɪs/ n. 假说

cell nucleus with **ultraviolet** light. Then he replaced the egg's nucleus with a nucleus from a specialized **intestinal** cell taken from a tadpole. If the specialized intestinal cell lacked important **segments** of the genetic material it would not be able to generate **tadpoles**. But it could — John B. Gurdon's **manipulated** frog's eggs gave rise to both **wriggling** tadpoles and full-grown frogs.

ultraviolet /ˌʌltrəˈvaɪələt/ adj. 紫外的
intestinal/ˌɪntesˈtaɪnl/ adj. 肠的
tadpole /ˈtædpəul/ n. 蝌蚪
segment /ˈsegmənt/ n. 一部分
manipulate /məˈnɪpjʊleɪt/ v. 控制
wriggle /ˈrɪgl/ v. 蠕动

6. John B. Gurdon demonstrated that the genetic material in the body's mature cells has the same potential as the genetic material in egg cells. With its help, it is possible to create all the **myriad** cells of the body—or a whole new individual. In other words, the cells still contained all the genetic information the researchers had previously believed was lost. But the genes are only activated if the nucleus is taken out and transferred into an empty egg cell. The **slumbering** potential of the adult nucleus is somehow awakened in the egg cell. Theoretically, it should be possible to **reprogram** the nucleus while it is still in the adult cell, but that would require more detailed knowledge about the **intrinsic mechanisms** that regulate cell development.

myriad /ˈmɪriəd/ n. 无数
slumber /ˈslʌmbə(r)/ v. 睡眠
reprogram /rɪˈprəʊgræm/ v. 重组
intrinsic /ɪnˈtrɪnsɪk/ adj. 固有的
mechanism /ˈmekənɪzəm/ n. 机制

Life there and back again

7. Shinya Yamanaka[2] was born in 1962, the same year John B. Gurdon reported the arrival of his cloned tadpoles. Forty-four years later, Yamanaka was to find a new recipe to reprogram cells, inspired both by John B. Gurdon's work and by modern stem cell

research. With this recipe in hand, he was the first to **induce** mature cells to **reverse** their development and turn back into stem cells.

induce /ɪn'dju:s/ v. 诱发
reverse /rɪ'vɜ:s/ v. 反转

8. Early in his career, Shinya Yamanaka dedicated himself to surgery and molecular biology, but he was soon attracted to the many possibilities of pluripotent stem cells. In his laboratory in Nara, Japan, he began to study embryonic stem cells — pluripotent cells that can be harvested from early embryos. He wanted to understand how they retain their pluripotency; in other words, he wanted to figure out what prevents them from developing into specialized cells.

9. One known characteristic of pluripotent cells was that a specific set of genes are active. These genes encode proteins called **transcription** factors, which in turn regulate other genes in the cell. When Shinya Yamanaka had succeeded in identifying yet another gene that was important for the pluripotency of embryonic stem cells, he believed he had the knowledge he needed. Now it was time to put it to the test.

transcription /træn'skrɪpʃn/ n. 转录

10. Instead of studying how stem cells are maintained as pluripotent cells, he started at the other end and tried to get specialized cells to turn back into stem cells. After selecting 24 of the genes that were associated with pluripotency, he and his co-workers inserted them into **fibroblast** cells from the skin of mice, one gene at a time, with the help of a virus. Nothing happened. But when he inserted all 24 genes at once, some of the

fibroblast /'faɪbrəblæst/ n. 纤维组织母细胞

cells started to change their shape: they **plumped up** and their nuclei grew. They were **converted** into something very similar to embryonic stem cells.

plump up /plʌmp ʌp/ v. 鼓起
convert /kən'vɜːt/ v. 转变

11. It was a groundbreaking discovery, but Shinya Yamanaka wanted to go even farther. He repeated the experiment over and over, gradually reducing the number of genes he inserted. Ultimately he found a surprisingly simple recipe: only four of the genes were required to get the fibroblasts to go into reverse and become pluripotent stem cells.

12. In later experiments, Shinya Yamanaka was able to demonstrate that the reversed cells—which he called iPS cells (induced pluripotent stem cells)—truly were pluripotent. The iPS cells that he injected into mouse embryos started to diversify into more specialized cells that contributed to the formation of all tissues in the adult mouse.

A technique with many possibilities

13. When Shinya Yamanaka published his findings in 2006 the scientific community paid very close attention. Before long, researchers all over the world had started experimenting with Yamanaka's simple basic recipe and soon the technique had developed in several ways.

14. One year later, Shinya Yamanaka and other researchers succeeded in generating iPS cells from human skin cells. This strengthened the hope that iPS cells might someday be used for medical purposes.

In the future scientists hope to be able to use iPS cells to **culture** cells that can be **transplanted** into the body and replace diseased cells.

culture /ˈkʌltʃə(r)/ v. 培养
transplant /trænsˈplɑːnt/ v. 移植

15. The iPS technique also means that researchers now have an unlimited source for stem cells. Stem cell research has relied heavily on embryonic stem cells harvested from embryos. Human embryos are not easy to come by, and many consider research involving use of human embryonic stem cells to be ethically questionable. Embryonic stem cells will continue to be of great scientific interest, but in many situations researchers can now use iPS cells instead. (1142 words)

Notes:

1. John B. Gurdon: 约翰•伯特兰•格登爵士，1933 年 10 月 2 日出生，是一位英国发育生物学家。他主要以在细胞核移植与克隆方面的先驱性研究而知名。
2. Shinya Yamanaka: 山中伸弥，日本医学家，1962 年出生于日本大阪府，毕业于大阪市立大学。现任京都大学 iPS 细胞研究所所长，美国加利福尼亚州旧金山心血管疾病研究所高级研究员。

Task 1: Reading Skills Practice

Directions: Read text B carefully and try to identify the organizational patterns in this article. Find detailed information about the methods used in the corresponding paragraphs. (See ***Skills Bank***)

Organizational patterns	Methods	Detailed information	Para.
explain and analyze	example/ illustration		

续表

Organizational patterns	Methods	Detailed information	Para.
explain and analyze	clarification		
	definition		
	division/ classification		
	cause/effect		
	compare/contrast		

Task 2: Text-related Presentation

Directions:Take turns to make a 1-min presentation about the following topics. Your presentation should be based on the text but not limited to the text. You are encouraged to present in a unique and creative way.

1) Introduce the analogy between life's one-way journey and cells' differentiation process in your own words. (Para.1-Para.3)

2) Draw up a profile of the Nobel laureate John B. Gurdon. You can include such elements as education, career choice, life, etc. (Para.4-Para.14)

3) Demonstrate John B. Gurdon's 1962 experiment by drawing pictures on the blackboard or showing the self-made pictures (Para.5)

4) Explain Shinya Yamanaka's experiment on iPS cells. (Para.10-Para.12)

5) Introduce the application of iPS technique. (Para.13-Para.15)

After You Read

Task 1: Oral Presenting

Directions: Try to rephrase or explain the following sentences without using the boldfaced words or phrases. (This is going to be integrated into the communicative interaction in the classroom. The task can be done orally in the classroom.)

1. If the specialized intestinal cell **lacked** important segments of the genetic material it **would not** be able to generate tadpoles.
2. The **slumbering** potential of the adult nucleus is somehow **awakened** in the

egg cell.

3. When Shinya Yamanaka had **succeeded in identifying** yet another gene that was important for the pluripotency of embryonic stem cells, he believed he had the knowledge he needed.
4. The iPS cells that he injected into mouse embryos started to **diversify into** more specialized cells that **contributed to** the formation of all tissues in the adult mouse.
5. Human embryos are not easy to come by, and many consider research involving use of human embryonic stem cells to be **ethically questionable.**

Task 2: Critical Thinking

Directions: Work in groups and discuss the following question. At the end of your discussion, each group will assign a representative to present your pints on this issue.

Stem cell research has the potential to dramatically alter approaches to understanding and treating diseases, and to alleviating suffering. However, the status of human embryonic stem cell research has always been under the spotlight. Why is it such a controversial issue? Do you support stem cell research regardless of any pro-life misgivings?

After-class Tasks

Task 1: Word Chunks

Directions: Complete the following word chunks taken from Text A and Text B according to their Chinese equivalents and make a sentence with each word chunk.

1. ________ molecule 合成细胞
2. muscle ________ 肌肉收缩
3. form ________ 形成基质
4. test ________ 试验假设
5. ________ iPS cell 产生多能干细胞
6. intrinsic ________ 内在机理
7. ________ embryo 获取胚胎
8. ________ fibroblast 反转纤维母细胞
9. ________ cell 特化细胞
10. ________ cell 反转细胞
11. ________ ovum 受精卵
12. ________ electric signal 引发电信号
13. ________ iPS cell 多功能的多能干细胞
14. ________ nucleus 重组细胞核
15. ________ mature cell 诱导成熟细胞
16. ________ protein 编码蛋白质
17. ________ genes 转移基因
18. ________ cells 培养细胞
19. ________ factor 转码因子
20. cell ________ 细胞衰退

Task 2: Translation

Directions: Translate sentence 1 to 3 into Chinese and pay close attention to the translation of the words in bold. Then translate sentence 4 to 6 into English using the words in the bracket.

1. There are three types of muscle cells-**skeletal, cardiac, and smooth-muscle cells**—all of which generate forces and produce movement but differ from each other in shape, in the mechanism controlling their **contractile activity**, and in their location in the various organs of the body.

____

____

2. This **matrix** may vary in consistency from a semifluid gel, in loose connective tissue, to the **solid crystallized structure of bone.**

____

____

3. These genes **encode proteins** called **transcription** factors, which in turn **regulate** other genes in the cell.

____

____

4. 神经细胞的活动构成了很多现象的基础，如意识、感知及认知。(underlie)

____

____

5. 只有取出细胞核并把其转移到一个空的卵细胞，基因才会被激活。(activate)

____

____

6. 目前，干细胞研究主要依赖从胚胎中获取的胚胎干细胞。(rely on)

____

____

Task 3: Listening & Speaking

Directions: Watch the video *Parkinson's disease—Progress and Promise in Stem Cell* and complete the following guided note-taking.

Word Bank

neuro-degenerative adj. 神经系统退化的
culture dish 培养皿
gait [geɪt] n. 步态
substantia nigra n. 黑质
stoop [stu:p] n. 驼背
irreparably[ɪ'repərəblɪ] adv. 不能挽回地

1. Recommended medication or therapies for Parkinson's disease

____

2. Explanation of substantia nigra

____

3. Mechanism of the application of iPS cells in the treatment of Parkinson's disease.

____

Task 4: Research

Directions: Do some research into *medical application of iPS cells and the challenges or limitations This New Cell Technology Faces*. You can present in the form of an interview, short play or simply a lecture. Make sure each member of the group will present his or her part on the stage. You can present in the form of an interview, short play or simply a lecture. Make sure each member of the group will present his or her part on the stage.

Resources

http://www.cira.kyoto-u.ac.jp/e/pressrelease/other/140227-140325.html
http://genesdev.cshlp.org/content/24/20/2239
http://hmg.oxfordjournals.org/content/early/2013/08/19/hmg.ddt379.full
http://stemcells.nih.gov/info/Regenerative_Medicine/pages/2006chapter10.aspx

Task 5: Writing

Directions: The cloning of humans is an ethical dilemma. Advocates claim that human cloning can generate tissues and whole organs to treat patients who cannot obtain transplants. However, opponents of cloning have concerns that technology is not yet developed enough to be safe. Write an essay titled ***My View on the Cloning of Humans.***

***Task* 6: Vocabulary Log**

Directions: Please finish the vocabulary log (Please find the log at the end of the book)by looking up the dictionary and write down the words or expressions you have learnt in this unit by following the examples already listed in the log. And then write down the translation for each vocabulary item and if possible, its variants, synonym, and the frequent collocations.

Task 7: Reading Log

Directions: After learning the whole unit and conducting the research, you have known more about cells from different perspectives. You can go to the library or surf on the internet for more knowledge about it. You can take down the key information according to the sample chart.(Please find the chart at the end of the book) Also you are allowed to complete the chart on a computer or tablet so that this section is expandable if you want to write more than the space on a paper form might allow. And then send it to your teacher by emails. The reading log can serve as an informal way to keep track of your reading progress.

Unit 3

Art of Medicine

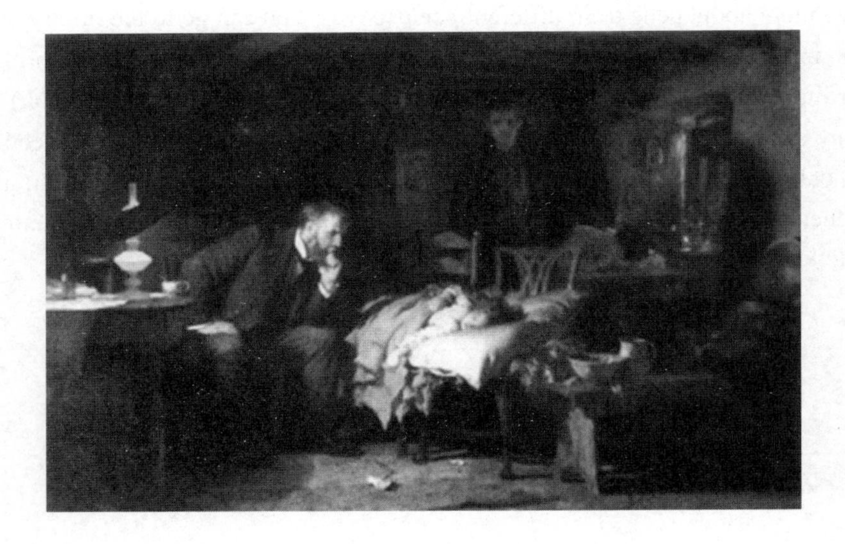

Wherever the art of medicine is loved, there is also a love of humanity"

——Hippocrates

Skills Bank

Recognizing Relationships Between Sentences

When you are recognizing relationships between sentences, you are identifying the ways authors connect their ideas between their sentences. Authors can explicitly tell you what this link is by using transition words. OR authors can implicitly link ideas in their sentences and the reader must figure out what the relationship is between the sentences.There are nine ways authors can create relationships between sentences.

1. Addition

In addition relationships, authors link elements between their sentences by adding more items and ideas without making one sentence dependent upon another. Transitional words: and, also, in addition...

2. Clarification

Clarification between sentences occurs when authors restate their point to promote understanding. Transitional words: be classified, to categorize...

3. Comparison

Authors make comparisons when two ideas or items have something in common. Transitional words: in the same way, similar to...

4. Contrast

Authors create a contrast between two sentences when these sentences display differences between them. One way of demonstrating a contrasting relationship is to use sentences that contradict one another. Transitional words: unlike, in contrast to...

5. Example

Authors include examples in their sentences to provide a more concrete instance of an idea, event, or general statement they have made. Transitional words: for example, for instance...

6. Location or Spatial Order

When authors relate one or more items or objects to each other or to the surrounding space, they are using location/spatial order. Transitional words: in front of, beside...

7. Cause and Effect

If one event precedes another event and results in a specific outcome, then the initial event is the "cause" and the specific outcome is the "effect." Transitional words: on account of, as a result...

8. Summary

Authors often use summary structure to condense the main points and essential elements of their passage. Transitional words: to summarize, to sum up

9. Time

There are two types of time relationship. Transitional words: first, second...

Pre-class Tasks

Task 1: Medical Terminology Study

Directions: Study the word roots, prefixes and suffixes listed in the table below and do the **Vocabulary Preview** exercise for Text A or/ and Text B according to your teacher's instructions.

Roots	Meaning
physi/o	relating to nature and living things 与自然、生理、物理有关的
iatr/o	of or pertaining to medicine, or a physician 医师，医学，医疗
bi/o	life 生物，生命
path/o	disease 病理
mort/o	death 死亡
my/o	of or relating to muscle 肌肉
cardi/o	of or pertaining to the heart 心，心脏
ventr/o	of or pertaining to the belly; the stomach cavities 腹，腹侧
rhythm/o	rhythm 节律，节奏
gnos/o	knowledge 知识
hom/o	the same 相同
chol/e	of or pertaining to bile 胆汁，胆
gluc/o	sweet 甘，甜，葡萄糖
pod/o	of or pertaining to foot 足，脚
oste/o	bone 骨

续表

Roots	Meaning
mamm/o	of or pertaining to the breast 乳房，乳腺
colon/o	colon 结肠
pneum/o	of or pertaining to the lungs 肺，呼吸，空气，气
neur/o	of or pertaining to nerves and the nervous system 神经
Prefixes	**Meaning**
sub-	beneath 不足，次，低于，分支，副，附属，亚
micro-	denoting something as small, or relating to smallness 微小
anti-	against 反，对抗，解，抑制，退，代替
multi-	many 多，多数，复
pre-	before; in front of 在前，先，在先，预先
re-	again, backward 再，复，回，重新
a-	not, without 不，无，缺，离
dia-	through, during, across 通过，透析，横
hyper-	extreme, beyond normal 超，超过，多，高，过多，上，重
Suffixes	**Meaning**
-genic	formative, pertaining to producing 产生，生产
-al	pertaining to… ……的
-genesis	producing, forming 起源，发生
-gen	substance that produces 发生，原
-rrhage	burst forth 出血，流血
-stasis	stopping, standing 固定，停滞，郁滞
-ose	sugar 糖，碳水化合物，蛋白质产物
-iatry	denotes a field in medicine of a certain body component 医疗术
-porosis	condition of pores 疏松
-gram	record or picture 表示书写物，图，像，记录，书写，图像
-scopy	use of instrument for viewing 观察，检查，检查法，镜检法

Task 2: Prepared Individual Presentation

Directions: The assigned students need to prepare a 1-min oral presentation concerning the questions in **Text-related Presentation** for Text A and/or Text B as required by your teacher.

Task 3: The Muddiest Points

Directions: Read Text A and Text B in the study group to find out the sentences that are the least clear to you after your discussions, the viewpoints that you disagree with and the understanding you have achieved through discussions and the questions you want to put forward concerning the content of the texts. Put the above information in a slip and send it to the teacher via WeChat 24 hours prior to the class. (The slip can be found on the last page of the book.)

In-class Tasks

Text A

Before You Read

Task 1: Vocabulary Preview

Directions: Divide the following words into their word parts and then give their Chinese translations by referring to **Medical Teminology Study**.

Medical Terms	Prefix	Word Root(s)	Suffix	Chinese
physiology				
iatrogenic				
microbial				
pathogenesis				
antigen				
multigenic				
presymptomatic				
myocardial				
arrhythmia				
mortality				
biology				
homogeneous				

Task 2: Warming-up

Directions: Watch the video carefully and try to answer the questions below. While watching the video, please take some notes in the blanks to help you to memorize the information.

1) The doctor is taking Physician's Oath. Do you know the history of the oath?
2) According to the oath, what will be doctors' number one consideration?
3) According to the oath, what should not be intervened between a doctor's duty and

the patient?

4) How should a doctor handle human rights and civil liberties?

Notes

Text A Approach to Medicine

1. Medicine is a profession that **incorporates** science and the scientific method with the art of being a physician. The art of tending to the sick is as old as humanity itself. Even in modern times, the art of caring and comforting,guided by millennia of common sense as well as a more recent, systematic approach to medical ethics, remains the **cornerstone** of medicine.Without these humanistic qualities, the application of the modern science of medicine is **suboptimal**, ineffective, or even **detrimental**.

2. The caregivers of ancient times and premodern cultures tried a variety of interventions to help the afflicted. Some of their potions contained what are now known to be active ingredients that form the basis for proven medications. Others have persisted into the present era despite a lack of convincing

incorporate /ɪnˈkɔːpəreɪt/ v. 把……合并

cornerstone /ˈkɔːnəstəʊn/ n. 基础

suboptimal /sʌbˈɔptiməl/ adj. 次最优的

detrimental /detrɪˈment(ə)l/ adj. 有害的

evidence. Modern medicine should not dismiss the possibility that these unproven approaches may be helpful;instead, it should adopt a guiding principle that all interventions, whether traditional or newly developed, can be tested vigorously, with the expectation that any beneficial effects can be explored further to determine their scientific basis.

3. When compared with its long and generally **distinguished** history of caring and comforting, the scientific basis of medicine is remarkably recent. Other than an understanding of human **anatomy** and the later description, albeit widely contested at this time, of the normal **physiology** of the circulatory system, almost all of modern medicine is based on discoveries made within the past 150 years. Until the late 19th century, the **paucity** of medical knowledge was perhaps exemplified best by hospitals and hospital care. Although hospitals provided caring that all but well-to-do people might not be able to obtain elsewhere, there is little if any evidence that hospitals improved health outcomes. The term hospitalism referred not to expertise in hospital care but rather to the **aggregate** of **iatrogenic** afflictions that were induced by the hospital stay itself.

4. Modern medicine has moved rapidly past organ physiology to an increasingly detailed understanding of cellular, subcellular, and genetic mechanisms.For example, the understanding of microbial pathogenesis and many **inflammatory** diseases is now guided

distinguished /dɪ'stɪŋgwɪʃt/ adj. 著名的

anatomy /ə'nætəmɪ/ n. 解剖；解剖学

physiology /ˌfɪzɪ'ɒlədʒɪ/ n. 生理学；生理机能

paucity /'pɔːsɪtɪ/ n. 缺乏

aggregate /'ægrɪgət/ n. 集合；合计

iatrogenic /aɪˌætrə(ʊ)'dʒenɪk/ adj. 医源性的

inflammatory /ɪn'flæmət(ə)rɪ/ adj. 炎症性的

by a detailed understanding of the human immune system and its response to foreign **antigens**.

antigen /ˈæntɪdʒ(ə)n/ n. 抗原

5. Health, disease, and an individual's interaction with the environment are also substantially determined by genetics. In addition to many conditions that may be determined by a single gene, medical science increasingly understands the complex interactions that underlie **multigenic** traits. In the not-so-distant future, the decoding of the human **genome** holds the promise that personalized health care can be targeted according to an individual's genetic profile, in terms of screening and presymptomatic disease management, as well as in terms of specific medications and their adjusted dosing schedules. Currently, knowledge of the structure and physical forms of proteins helps explain abnormalities as diverse as **sickle** cell **anemia**[1] and prion-related diseases. Proteomics,which is the normal and abnormal protein expression of genes, also holds extraordinary promise for developing drug targets for more specific and effective therapies.

multigenic /ˌmʌltɪˈdʒiːnɪk/ adj. 多基因的

genome /ˈdʒiːnəʊm/ n. 基因组

sickle /ˈsɪk(ə)l/ n. 镰刀

anemia /əˈniːmɪə/ n. 贫血；贫血症

6. Concurrent with these advances in fundamental human biology has been a dramatic shift in methods for evaluating the application of scientific advances to the individual patient and to populations. The randomized controlled trial, sometimes with thousands of patients at multiple institutions, has replaced **anecdote** as the preferred method

anecdote /ˈænɪkdəʊt/ n. 轶事

for measuring the benefits and optimal uses of diagnostic and therapeutic interventions. As studies progress from those that show biologic effect, to those that elucidate dosing schedules and **toxicity**, and finally to those that assess true clinical benefit, the metrics of measuring outcome has also improved from subjective impressions of physicians or patients to reliable and valid measures of **morbidity**, quality of life, functional status, and other patient-oriented outcomes. These marked improvements in the scientific methodology of clinical investigation have expedited extraordinary changes in clinical practice, such as recanalization therapy[2] for acute **myocardial infarction**[3], and have shown that reliance on intermediate outcomes, such as a reduction in **asymptomatic ventricular arrhythmias**[4] with certain drugs, may unexpectedly increase rather than decrease **mortality**. Just as physicians in the 21st century must understand advances in fundamental biology, similar understanding of the fundamentals of clinical study design as it applies to diagnostic and therapeutic interventions is needed. An understanding of human genetics will also help stratify and refine the approach to clinical trials by helping researchers select fewer patients with a more **homogeneous** disease pattern to study the efficacy of an intervention.

7. This explosion in medical knowledge has led to increasing specialization and subspecialization, defined initially by organ

toxicity /tɒkˈsɪsətɪ/ n. 毒性

morbidity /mɔːˈbɪdətɪ/ n. 发病率

myocardial/ˌmaɪəʊˈkɑːdɪəl/ adj. 心肌的

infarction /ɪnˈfɑːkʃ(ə)n/ n. 梗塞

asymptomatic /əˌsɪmptəˈmætɪk/ adj. 无症状的

ventricular /venˈtrɪkjʊlə/ adj. 心室的

arrhythmia /eɪˈrɪðmɪə/ n. 心律不齐

mortality /mɔːˈtælɪtɪ/ n. 死亡率

homogeneous/ˌhɒmə(ʊ)ˈdʒiːnɪəs/ adj. 同种类的

system and more recently by locus of principal activity (**inpatient** vs. **outpatient**), reliance on manual skills(proceduralist vs. non-proceduralist), or participation in research. Nevertheless,it is becoming increasingly clear that the same fundamental **molecular** and genetic mechanisms are broadly applicable across all organ systems and that the scientific methodologies of randomized trials and careful clinical observation span all aspects of medicine.

inpatient /ˈɪnpeɪʃnt/ n. 住院病人

outpatient /ˈaʊtpeɪʃ(ə)nt/ n. 门诊病人

molecular /məˈlekjʊlə/ adj. 分子的

8. The advent of modern approaches to managing data now provides the **rationale** for the use of health information technology. Computerized health records, oftentimes shared with patients in a portable format, can avoid duplication of tests and assure that care is coordinated among the patient's various health care providers. (855 words)

rationale /ˌræʃəˈnɑːl/ n. 基本原理

Notes:

1. sickle cell anemia: 镰状细胞贫血。主要见于非洲下撒哈拉地区出生的居民及其后裔，以及中东、地中海地区和印度。异常的血红蛋白将红血球扭曲成坚硬的镰刀形状。临床表现为慢性溶血性贫血、易感染和再发性疼痛危象以致慢性局部缺血导致器官组织损害。
2. incarnation therapy: 再通疗法。在机化过程中，因血栓逐渐干燥收缩，其内部或与血管壁间出现裂隙，新生的内皮细胞长入并被覆其表面，形成迷路状的通道，血栓上下游的血流得以部分恢复，这种现象称为再通。
3. myocardial infarction: 心肌梗死。是冠状动脉急性、持续性缺血缺氧所引起的心肌坏死。临床上多有剧烈而持久的胸骨后疼痛，休息及硝酸酯类药物不能完全缓解，伴有血清心肌酶活性增高及进行性心电图变化，可并发心律失常、休克或心力衰竭，常可危及生命。

4. ventricular arrhythmia: 室性心律失常指起源于心室的心律紊乱。常见的心律失常包括室性早搏（室早）、室性心动过速（室速）、心室颤动（室颤）等。

While You Read

Task 1: Text-related Presentation

Directions:Take turns to make a 1-min presentation about the following topics. Your presentation should be based on the text but not limited to the text. You are encouraged to present in a unique and creative way.

1) Talk about the art of tending to the sick is in old times. (Para. 1)

2) Explain why the modern medicine is based on discoveries made within the past 150 years. (Para. 3)

3) List and describe the approaches of modern medicine (Para. 5- Para. 7)

4) Describe the specialization and subspecialization in medicine. (Para. 7)

5) Describe how computerized health records avoid duplication of tests and assure that care is coordinated among the patient's various health care providers. (Para. 8)

After You Read

Task 1: Academic English Study

Directions: Read this section carefully and try to find more examples of nominal group from Text A and Text B.

Complexity (I)

Nominal Groups

Academic written English uses nouns and nominal group (noun-based phrases) more than verbs. It is lexically dense — there is a higher proportion of content words per clause. This can be done by modification of nouns to form nominal groups.

A typical nominal group is structured in the following way:

determiner	premodifier	head	postmodifier
a	complicated	solution	to the problem

One simple example is:

Like all other forms of life, we human beings are the product of *evolution*.

Like all other forms of life, we human beings are the product of *how we have evolved.*

The noun "evolution" is preferred to the verb "evolve" and the "wh" clause.

Ex1: Without these humanistic qualities, the *application* of the modern science of medicine is suboptimal, ineffective, or even detrimental. (Para 1)

Ex2: The *advent* of modern approaches to managing data now provides the rationale for the *use* of health information technology. (Para 8)

Task 2: Critical Thinking

Directions: Work in groups and discuss the following question. At the end of your discussion, each group will assign a representative to present your opinions on this issue.

How do you understand "Without humanistic qualities, the application of the modern science of medicine is suboptimal, ineffective, or even detrimental."? Can you use some examples to illustrate your understanding?

Text B

Before You Read

Task 1: Vocabulary Preview

Directions: Preview the words in the table below and use them to describe the following pictures.

microbial antigen myocardial arrhythmia pathogenesis recanalization

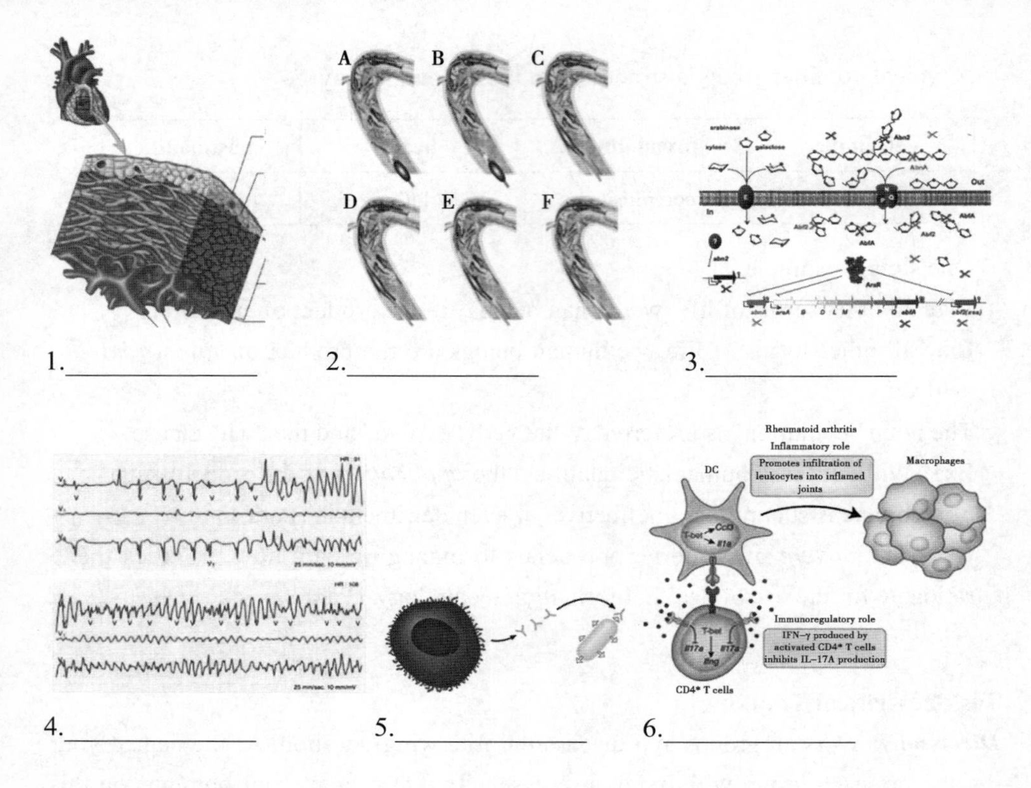

1.______________ 2.______________ 3.______________

4.______________ 5.______________ 6.______________

Task 2: Warming-up

Directions: Watch the video carefully and try to answer the questions below. While watching the video, please take some notes in the blanks to help you to memorize the information.

1) Why does the doctor feel sorry for his patient?

2) According to the lecture, what can make a good doctor?

Notes

Text B Neuron Overload and the Juggling Physician

Danielle Ofri

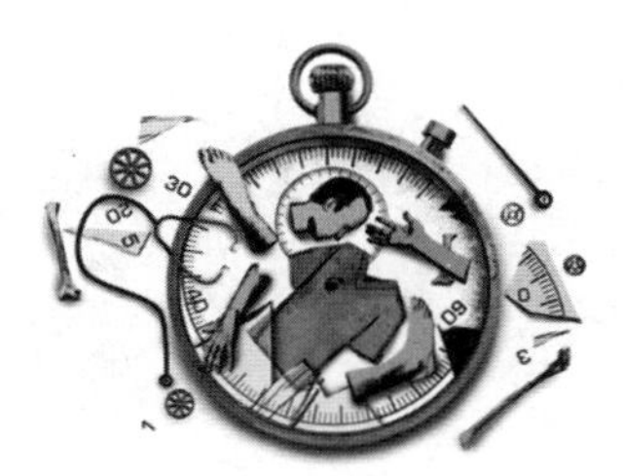

1. Patients often complain that their doctors don't listen. Although there are probably a few doctors who truly are tone-deaf, most are reasonably **empathic** human beings, and I wonder why even these doctors seem prey to this criticism. I often wonder whether it is sheer **neuron** overload on the doctor side that leads to this problem. Sometimes it feels as though my brain is juggling so many competing details, that one stray request from a patient—even one that is quite relevant—might send the delicately balanced three-ring circus tumbling down.

empathic /em'pæθɪk/ adj. 移情作用的

neuron /'njʊərɒn/ n. 神经元，神经细胞

2. One day, I tried to work out how many details a doctor needs to keep spinning in her head in order to do a satisfactory job, by calculating how many thoughts I have to juggle in a typical office visit. Mrs. Osorio is a 56-year-old woman in my practice. She is somewhat overweight. She has reasonably well-controlled **diabetes** and **hypertension**. Her **cholesterol** is on the high side but she doesn't take any medications for this. She

diabetes /ˌdaɪə'biːtiːz/ n. 糖尿病

hypertension /haɪpə'tenʃ(ə)n/ n. 高血压

cholesterol /kə'lestərɒl/ n. 胆固醇

doesn't exercise as much as she should, and her last DEXA scan[1] showed some thinning of her bones. She describes her life as stressful, although she's been good about keeping her appointments and getting her blood tests. She's generally healthy, someone who'd probably be described as an average patient in a medical practice, not excessively complicated. Here are the thoughts that run through my head as I proceed through our 20-min **consultation**.

3. Good thing she did her blood tests. **Glucose** is a little better. Cholesterol isn't great. May need to think about starting a **statin**. Are her liver **enzymes** normal? Her weight is a little up. I need to give her my talk about five fruits and vegetables and 30 min of walking each day. Diabetes: how do her morning sugars compare to her evening sugars? Has she spoken with the **nutritionist** lately? Has she been to the eye doctor? The **podiatrist**? Her blood pressure is good but not great. Should I add another BP med? Will more pills be confusing? Does the benefit of possible better blood pressure control outweigh the risk of her possibly not taking all of her meds? Her bones are a little thin on the DEXA. Should I start a bisphosphonate[2] that might prevent **osteoporosis**? But now I'm piling yet another pill onto her, and one that requires detailed instructions. Maybe leave this until next time? How are things at home? Is she experiencing just the usual stress of life, or might there be depression or anxiety disorder **lurking**? Is

consultation /kɒnsəl'teɪʃ(ə)n/ n. 会诊；讨论会

glucose /'gluːkəʊs; -z/ n. 葡萄糖

statin /'stætɪn/ n. 他汀类，抑制素

enzyme /'enzaɪm/ n. 酶

nutritionist /njʊ'trɪʃ(ə)nɪst/ n. 营养学家

podiatrist /pə'daɪətrɪst/ n. 足病医生

osteoporosis /ˌɒstɪəʊpə'rəʊsɪs/ n. 骨质疏松症

lurk /lɜːk/ v. 潜伏，潜藏，埋伏

there time for the depression questionnaire? Health maintenance: when was her last mammogram[3]? PAP **smear**? Has she had a **colonoscopy** since she turned 50? Has she had a **tetanus** booster in the past 10 years? Does she qualify for a **pneumonia** vaccine?

smear /smɪə/ n. 涂片
colonoscopy /ˌkəʊlə'nɒskəpɪ/ n. 结肠镜检查
tetanus /'tet(ə)nəs/ n. 破伤风
pneumonia /njuː'məʊnɪə/ n. 肺炎

4. Ms Osorio interrupts my train of thought to tell me that her back has been aching for the past few months. From her perspective, this is probably the most important item in our visit, but the fact is that she's caught one of my neurons in mid-fire (the one that's thinking about her blood sugar, which is **segueing** into the neuron that's preparing the diet-and-exercise discussion, which is intersecting with the one that's debating about initiating a statin). My instinct is to put one hand up and keep all interruptions at bay. It's not that I don't want to hear what she has to say, but the sensation that I'm juggling so many thoughts, and need to resolve them all before the clock runs down, that keeps me in moderate state of panic. What if I drop one—what if one of my thoughts **evaporates** while I address another concern? I'm trying to type as fast as I can, for the very sake of not letting any thoughts escape, but every time I turn to the computer to write, I'm not making eye contact with Mrs Osorio. I don't want my patient to think that the computer is more important than she is, but I have to keep looking toward the screen to get her lab results, check her mammogram report, document the progress of her illnesses, order the tests, refill her prescriptions.

segue /'segweɪ/ n. 继续（用作指示语）
evaporate /ɪ'væpəreɪt/ v. 蒸发

5. Then she pulls a form out of her bag: her insurance company needs this form for some reason or another. An innocent—and completely justified—request, but I feel that this could be the straw that breaks the camel's back, that the precarious balance of all that I'm keeping in the air will be simply unhinged. I nod, but indicate that we need to do her physical examination first. I barrel through the basics, then quickly check for any red-flag signs that might suggest that her back pain is anything more than routine muscle strain. I return to the computer to input all the information, mentally running though my checklist, anxious that nothing important slips from my brain's holding bay.

6. I want to do everything properly and cover all our bases, but the more effort I place into accurate and thorough documentation, the less time I have to actually interact with my patient. A glance at the clock tells me that we've gone well beyond our allotted time. I stand up and hand Mrs. Osorio her prescriptions. "What about my insurance form," she asks. "It needs to be in by Friday, otherwise I might lose my coverage." I clap my hand against my forehead; I've completely forgotten about the form she'd asked about just a few minutes ago.

7. Studies have **debunked** the myth of multitasking in human beings. The concept of multitasking was developed in the computer field to explain the idea of a microprocessor doing two jobs at one time. It turns out that

debunk /diːˈbʌŋk/ v. 揭穿

microprocessors are in fact linear, and actually perform only one task at a time. Our computers give the illusion of simultaneous action based on the microprocessor "scheduling" competing activities in a complicated integrated **algorithm**. Like microprocessors, we humans can't actually concentrate on two thoughts at the same exact time. We merely zip back and forth between them, generally losing accuracy in the process. At best, we can juggle only a handful of thoughts in this manner.

algorithm /ˈælgərɪð(ə)m/ n. 算法，运算法则

8. The more thoughts we juggle, the less we are able to attune fully to any given thought. To me, this is a recipe for disaster. Today I only forgot an insurance company form. But what if I'd forgotten to order her mammogram, or what if I'd refilled only five of her six medicines? What if I'd forgotten to fully explain the side-effects of one of her medications? The list goes on, as does the anxiety.

9. At the end of the day, my mind spins as I try to remember if I've forgotten anything. Mrs. Osorio had seven medical issues to consider, each of which required at least five separate thoughts: that's 35 thoughts. I saw ten patients that afternoon: that's 350. I'd supervised five residents that morning, each of whom saw four patients, each of whom generated at least ten thoughts. That's another 200 thoughts. It's not to say that we can't handle 550 thoughts in a working day, but each of these thoughts potentially carries great risk if improperly

evaluated. If I do a good job juggling 98% of the time, that still leaves ten thoughts that might get lost in the process. Any one of those lost thoughts could translate into a disastrous outcome, not to mention a possible lawsuit. Most doctors are reasonably competent, caring individuals, but the overwhelming swirl of thoughts that we must keep track of leaves many of us in a perpetual panic that something serious might slip. This is what keeps us awake at night.

10. There are many proposed solutions—computer-generated reminders, case managers, **ancillary** services. To me, the simplest one would be time. If I had an hour for each patient, I'd be a spectacular doctor. If I could let my thoughts roll linearly and singularly, rather than **simultaneously** and haphazardly, I wouldn't fear losing anything. I suspect that it would actually be more efficient, as my patients probably wouldn't have to return as frequently. But realistically, no one is going to hand me a golden hour for each of my patients. My choices seem to boil down to entertaining fewer thoughts, accepting decreased accuracy for each thought, giving up on thorough documentation, or having a constant headache from neuronal overload.

ancillary /æn'sɪlərɪ/ adj. 辅助的

simultaneously /ˌsɪml'teɪnɪəslɪ/ adv. 同时地

11. These are the choices that practicing physicians face every day, with every patient. Mostly we rely on our clinical judgment to prioritize, accepting the trade-off that is inevitable with any compromise. We attend to the medical issues that carry the greatest

weight and then have to let some of the lesser ones slide, with the hope that none of these seemingly lesser ones masks something grave.

12. Some computers have indeed achieved the goal of true multitasking, by virtue of having more than one microprocessor. In practice, that is like possessing an additional brain that can function independently and thus truly simultaneously. Unless the transplant field advances drastically, there is little hope for that particular *deus ex machina*. In some cases, having a dedicated and competent clinical partner such as a one-on-one nurse can come close to simulating a second brain, but most medical budgets don't allow for such staffing indulgence.(1649 words)

Notes:

1. DEXA scan: Dual Energy X Ray Absorptiometry scan 双能X线吸收扫描，双能X线吸收测量法技术采用X线球管作为射线源，产生两种不同能量的X线以消除软组织的影响，因而具有扫描时间短、分辨率高、检查精确度高、射线投照量小等特点，现已取代DPA而成为骨密度测定的常用方法。
2. bisphosphonate: 二磷酸盐
3. mammogram: 乳房X线照片，是一种应用放射线检查乳房病变的技术。有钼靶摄片和干板摄片两种，均适合观察软组织的结构。诊断乳癌的准确率可高达90%，也可用作乳腺癌高发人群中的普查。

While You Read

Task 1: Reading Skills Practice

Directions: Please write down the appropriate transitional words or phrases to create relationships between sentences by referring to the ***Skills Bank.***

1. She describes her life as stressful, _______ she's been good about keeping her appointments and getting her blood tests.

2. It's not that I don't want to hear what she has to say, but the sensation that I'm juggling so many thoughts, _______ need to resolve them all before the clock runs down, that keeps me in moderate state of panic.
3. I'm trying to type as fast as I can, _______ the very sake of not letting any thoughts escape, but every time I turn to the computer to write, I'm not making eye contact with Mrs Osorio.
4. I don't want my patient to think that the computer is more important than she is, _______ I have to keep looking toward the screen to get her lab results, check her mammogram report, document the progress of her illnesses, order the tests, refill her prescriptions.
5. _______ microprocessors, we humans can't actually concentrate on two thoughts at the same exact time.
6. Any one of those lost thoughts could translate into a disastrous outcome, _______ a possible lawsuit.
7. If I could let my thoughts roll linearly and singularly, _______ simultaneously and haphazardly, I wouldn't fear losing anything.
8. I suspect that it would actually be more efficient, _______ my patients probably wouldn't have to return as frequently.
9. _______ the transplant field advances drastically, there is little hope for that particular deus ex machina.
10. _______, having a dedicated and competent clinical partner such as a one-on-one nurse can come close to simulating a second brain, but most medical budgets don't allow for such staffing indulgence.

Task 2: Text-related Presentation

Directions:Take turns to make a 1-min presentation about the following topics. Your presentation should be based on the text but not limited to the text. You are encouraged to present in a unique and creative way.

1) List the factors that make patients believe that their doctors don't listen. (Para.1)

2) Describe Mrs Osorio's conditions. (Para. 2-Para.3)

3) Give a brief introduction of diabetes. (Para. 4- Para. 6)

4) Introduce the concept of multitasking. (Para.7)

5) List the possible solutions for physicians to handle the neuron overload. (Para. 9-11)

After You Read

Task 1: Oral Presenting

Directions: Try to rephrase or explain the following sentences without using the bold faced words or phrases. (This is going to be integrated into the communicative interaction in the classroom. The task can be done orally in the classroom.)

1. I often **wonder** whether it is sheer neuron **overload** on the doctor side that **leads to** this problem.
2. Sometimes it feels **as though** my brain is **juggling** so many **competing details**, that one **stray request** from a patient — even one that is quite relevant — might send the **delicately balanced** three-ring circus **tumbling down**.
3. An **innocent** — and completely justified — request, but I feel that this could be the **straw that breaks the camel's back**, that the **precarious balance** of all that I'm keeping in the air will be simply **unhinged**.
4. Mostly we rely on our clinical judgment to **prioritize**, accepting the **trade-off** that is inevitable with any compromise.
5. We attend to the medical issues that **carry the greatest weight** and then have to **let some of the lesser ones slide**, with the hope that none of these seemingly lesser ones **masks something grave**.

Task 2: Critical Thinking

Directions: Work in groups and discuss the following questions. At the end of your discussion, each group will assign a representative to present your pints on this issue. In recent years, doctor-patient relationships have come under the media spotlight in China after a number of high-profile, violent incidents at hospitals. What do you think is the root cause of all the anger? What changes are needed to make it more harmonious for both medical professionals and patients?

After-class Tasks

Task 1: Word Chunks

Directions: Complete the following word chunks taken from Text A and Text B according to their Chinese equivalents and make a sentence with each word chunk.

1. _______ the sick 照顾病人
2. _______ down 倒塌
3. _______ the modern science 现代科学的应用
4. genetic _______ 遗传机制
5. health care _______ 医疗服务人员
6. human _______ 人类免疫系统
7. _______ antigen 外源抗原
8. _______ future 不远的未来
9. dramatic _______ 戏剧性的转变
10. _______ trial 临床试验
11. _______ trial 随机试验
12. _______ overweight 有点超重
13. _______ diabetes 糖尿病得到好的控制
14. _______ of the bone 骨质减少
15. take _______ 服药
16. _______ of thought 思路
17. _______ the prescription 补充处方
18. _______ examination 体格检查
19. muscle _______ 肌肉拉伤
20. _______ a lawsuit 更不用说诉讼

Task 2: Translation

Directions: Translate sentence 1 to 3 into Chinese and pay close attention to the translation of words in bold. Then translate sentence 4 to 6 into English using the words in the bracket.

1. Without these humanistic qualities, the application of the modern science of medicine is **suboptimal**, ineffective, or even **detrimental**.

____

____

2. For example, the understanding of microbial pathogenesis and many inflammatory diseases is now guided by a detailed understanding of the human immune system and its response to **foreign antigens**.

____

____

3. I don't want my patient to think that the computer is more important than she is, but I have to keep looking toward the screen to get her lab results, check her mammogram report, document the progress of her illnesses, order the tests, **refill her prescriptions**.

____

____

4. 健康，疾病和个体与环境的相互作用也基本由遗传学决定。(be determined by)

____

____

5. 现在，现代管理数据方法的出现提供了使用健康信息技术的基本原理。(rationale)

____

____

6. 大多数医生都是相当有能力、有爱心的，但是因为我们必须跟踪过多的想法，这就使得许多医生永远恐慌、害怕一些重要的事情可能被我们所忽略。(overwhelming)

____

____

Task 3: Listening & Speaking

Directions: Watch the video and answer the following questions before you make an oral summary of what have heard from the video.

Word Bank

angiogenesis /ˌændʒɪə(ʊ)ˈdʒenɪsɪs/ n. 血管生成 myriad /ˈmɪrɪəd/ n. 无数
arthritis /ɑːˈθraɪtɪs/ n. 关节炎
Alzheimer's disease /ˈæltshaiməz/ 阿尔茨海默病
denominator /dɪˈnɒmɪneɪtə/ n. 分母；命名者

1. In what situations is angiogenesis out of balance?
2. What problems can insufficient angiogenesis lead to?
3. What disease can be driven by excessive angiogenesis?
4. What kind of realization is allowing the lecturer to reconceptualize the way that they actually approach many diseases by controlling angiogenesis?

Note Taking

Task 4: Research

Directions: Interview doctors from different specialties and get to know their daily work, and then brainstorm the following aspects in groups before you develop your discussions into an oral presentation for the next class. You can present in the form of an interview, short play or simply a lecture. Make sure each member of the group will present his or her part on the stage.

1) How many different tasks should a doctor do each day?

2) How do the doctors you interview handle their busy work?

3) Describe the relationship between doctors and patients according to the interview?

4) How's the condition in western countries?

Resources

Here are the websites where you can find the useful information for your research.

http://en.wikipedia.org/wiki/Doctor-patient_relationship

http://www.ncbi.nlm.nih.gov/pmc/articles/PMC1496871/

http://www.changesurfer.com/Hlth/DPReview.html

Task 5: Writing

Directions: Burnout is a common phenomenon among physicians. It can affect both doctors and patients in many negative ways. And the reasons behind can vary. Please do some research on the internet and make a survey among physicians in the nearby hospitals. Then report what you have found under the title ***Burnout of Physicians.***

Task 6: Vocabulary Log

Directions: Please finish the vocabulary log (Please find the log at the end of the book) by looking up the dictionary and write down the words or expressions you have learnt in this unit by following the examples already listed in the log. And then write down the translation for each vocabulary item and if possible, its variants, synonym, antonym and the frequent collocations.

Task 7: Reading Log

Directions: After learning the whole unit and conducting the research, you have known more about physicians from different perspectives. You can go to the library or surf on the internet for more knowledge about it. You can take down the key information according to the sample chart. (Please find the chart at the end of the book) Also you are allowed to complete the chart on a computer or tablet so that this section is expandable if you want to write more than the space on a paper form might allow. And then send it to your teacher by emails. The reading log can serve as an informal way to keep track of your reading progress.

Unit 4

Craftsmanship of Physicians

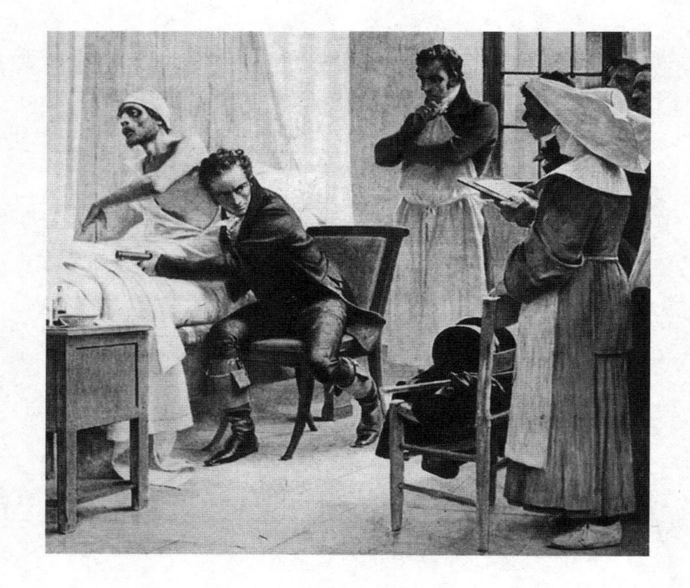

Medicine is learned by the bedside and not in the classroom.

——Sir William Osler

Skills Bank

Recognizing Relationships Within Sentences

When you are recognizing relationships within sentences, you are identifying the ways authors connect the ideas within their sentences. Authors can explicitly tell you what this link is by using transition words. OR authors can implicitly link ideas in their sentences and the reader must figure out what the relationship is.There are nine ways:

1. Addition

Authors link elements within their sentences by adding more items and ideas in addition relationships. Elements joined together in a series are examples of addition relationships.

2. Clarification

Clarification within a sentence occurs when authors restate their point to promote understanding.

3. Comparison

Authors make comparisons when two ideas or items have something in common. The author joins these two ideas or items so the reader recognizes the similarities between them.

4. Contrast

Authors contrast elements within sentences when the elements have differences between them.

5. Example

Authors include examples in their sentences to provide a more concrete instance of an idea, event, or general statement they have made.

6. Location or Spatial Order

When authors relate one or more items or objects to each other or to the surrounding space, they are using location/spatial order.

7. Cause and Effect

In cause and effect sentences, one part of the sentence is the source and one part is the outcome. For a sentence to use cause and effect structure, the cause must logically precede the effect!

8. Summary

Authors often use summary structure to condense the main points and essential elements of their passage.

9. Time

There are two types of time relationships.

Pre-class Tasks

Task 1: Medical Terminology Study

Directions: Study the word roots, prefixes and suffixes listed in the table below and do the **Vocabulary Preview** exercise for Text A or / and Text B according to your teacher's instructinstructions.

Roots	**Meaning**
inflect	vary the pitch of one's speech 音调变化
hepat/o	liver 肝
lip/o	fat 脂
tom/o	to cut 切割
tox	poison 毒
angi/o	vessal (blood)血管
nas/o	nose 鼻
cardi/o	heart 心脏
embol	embolus 栓子
neur/o	nerve 神经
steth/o	chest 胸
ophthalm/o	eye 眼
Prefixes	**Meaning**
a-	no; not; without 非
hyper-	having a lot or too much of a particular quality 过度
para-	beside; near 旁边
ultra-	beyond 超过的
iso-	equal or identical 相同，相等
endo-	in; within 内

续表

Prefixes	Meaning
intra-	within; inside 在内
sub-	under 下
Suffixes	**Meaning**
-pathy	feeling, sensitivity, or perception 感觉
-ism	a disease 病态
-ancy	a state 状况
-graphy	process of recording 记录法
-oma	tumor 肿瘤
-megaly	enlargement 扩大
-scope	instrument for visual examination 观察用仪器

Task 2: Prepared Individual Presentation

Directions: The assigned students need to prepare a 1-min oral presentation concerning the questions in **Text-related Presentation** for Text A and/or Text B as required by your teacher.

Task 3: The Muddiest Points

Directions: Read Text A and Text B in the study group to find out the sentences that are the least clear to you after your discussions, the viewpoints that you disagree with and the understanding you have achieved through discussions and the questions you want to put forward concerning the content of the texts. Put the above information in a slip and send it to the teacher via WeChat 24 hours prior to the class. (The slip can be found on the last page of the book.)

In-class Tasks

Text A

Before You Read

Task 1: Vocabulary Preview

Directions: Divide the following words into their word parts and then give their Chinese translations by referring to **Medical Terminology Study**.

Medical Terms	Prefix	Word Root(s)	Suffix	Chinese
abnormality				
hepatic				
hyperparathyroidism				
malignancy				
lipoprotein				
ultrasonography				
isotopic				
tomography				
nasolabial				
cadiomegaly				
endocarditis				
neurofibroma				
parasternal				

Task 2: Warming-up

Directions: Watch the video carefully and try to answer the questions below. While watching the video, please take notes in the blanks to help you follow the content.

1) According to the video, what is the main problem and the current situation?

2) Can you briefly describe the study mentioned in the video?

Notes

Text A Clinical Skills

1. The written history of an illness should include all the facts of medical significance in the life of the patient. Recent events should be given the most attention. The patient should, at some early point, have the opportunity to tell his or her own story of the illness without frequent interruption and, when appropriate, receive expressions of interest, encouragement, and **empathy** from the physician. Any event related by the patient, however **trivial** or seemingly irrelevant, may provide the key to solving the medical problem. In general, only patients who feel comfortable with the physician will offer complete information and thus **putting** the patient **at ease** to the greatest extent possible contributes substantially to obtaining an adequate history.

empathy /ˈempəθi/ n. 移情作用

trivial /ˈtrɪvɪəl/ adj. 不重要的，琐碎的

put...at ease 使不紧张，使安心

2. An informative history is more than an orderly listing of symptoms; by listening to patients and noting the way in which they describe their symptoms, physicians can gain valuable insight into the problem. **Inflections** of voice, facial expression, gestures, and attitude, i.e., "body language," may reveal important clues to the meaning of the symptoms to the patient. Because patients vary in their medical sophistication and ability to recall facts, the reported medical history should be **corroborated** whenever possible. The social history also can provide important

inflection /ɪnˈflekʃn/ n. 音调变化

corroborate /kəˈrɒbəreɪt/ v. 证实

insights into the types of diseases that should be considered. The family history not only identifies rare Mendelian disorders[1] within a family but often reveals risk factors for common disorders, such as coronary heart disease, hypertension, and asthma. A thorough family history may require input from multiple relatives to ensure completeness and accuracy, and once recorded, it can be updated readily. The process of history-taking provides an opportunity to observe the patient's behavior and watch for features to be pursued more thoroughly during the physical examination.

Physical examination

3. The purpose of the physical examination is to identify the physical signs of disease. The significance of these objective indications of disease is enhanced when they confirm a functional or structural change already suggested by the patient's history. At times, however, the physical signs may be the only evidence of disease.

4. The physical examination should be performed **methodically** and thoroughly, with consideration for the patient's comfort and modesty. Although attention is often directed by the history to the diseased organ or part of the body, the examination of a new patient must extend from head to toe in an objective search for **abnormalities**. Unless the physical examination is systematic and is performed in a consistent manner from patient to patient, important segments may be omitted **inadvertently**. The results of the examination,

methodically /mə'θɒdɪklɪ/ adv. 有系统地

abnormality /ˌæbnɔː'mæləti/ n. 异常

inadvertently /ˌɪnəd'vɜːtəntli/ adv. 出于无心的，由疏忽造成的

like the details of the history, should be recorded at the time they are **elicited**, not hours later, when they **are subject to** the distortions of memory. Skill in physical diagnosis is acquired with experience, but it is not merely technique that determines success in eliciting signs of disease. The detection of a few **scattered petechiae**, a faint **diastolic** murmur, or a small mass in the abdomen is not a question of keener eyes and ears or more sensitive fingers but of a mind alert to those findings. Because physical findings can change with time, the physical examination should be repeated as frequently as the clinical situation warrants. Because a large number of highly sensitive diagnostic tests are available, particularly imaging techniques, it may be tempting to **put** less **emphasis on** the physical examination.

elicit /ɪ'lɪsɪt/ v. 引出
be subject to 常遭受……
scattered /'skætəd/ adj. 分散的
petechiae /pə'tekɪeɪt/ n. 瘀点
diastolic /ˌdaɪə'stɒlɪk/ adj. 心脏舒张的
put emphasis on 强调

Diagnostic studies

5. Physicians have become increasingly reliant on **a** wide **array of** laboratory tests to solve clinical problems. **By virtue of** their impersonal quality, complexity, and apparent precision, laboratory tests often gain an **aura** of authority regardless of the **fallibility** of the tests, the instruments used in the tests, and the individuals performing or interpreting them.

6. Single laboratory tests are rarely ordered. Instead, physicians generally request "batteries" of multiple tests, which often prove useful. For example, abnormalities of **hepatic** function may provide the clue to nonspecific symptoms such as generalized

an array of 一批，大量
by virtue of 由于，凭借
aura /'ɔːrə/ n. 光环
fallibility /ˌfælə'bɪlətɪ/ n. 出错性
hepatic /hɪ'pætɪk/ adj. 肝的

weakness and increased **fatigability**, suggesting the diagnosis of chronic liver disease. Sometimes a single abnormality, such as an elevated **serum calcium** level, points to a particular disease, such as hyperparathyroidism[2] or an underlying **malignancy**.

7. The thoughtful use of screening tests such as low-density **lipoprotein** cholesterol may be quite useful. A group of laboratory determinations can be carried out conveniently on a single specimen at relatively low cost. Screening tests are most informative when directed toward common diseases or disorders and when their results indicate the need for other useful tests or interventions that may be costly to perform.

8. The development of technically improved imaging studies with greater sensitivity and **specificity** is one of the most rapidly advancing areas of medicine. These tests provide remarkably detailed anatomic information that can be a **pivotal** factor in medical decision-making. Ultrasonography[3], a variety of **isotopic** scans, CT, MRI, and **positron** emission tomography[4] have benefited patients by **supplanting** older, more invasive approaches and opening new diagnostic **vistas**. In light of their capabilities and the rapidity with which they can lead to a diagnosis, it is tempting to order **a battery of** imaging studies. All physicians have had experiences in which imaging studies turned up findings that led to an unexpected

fatigability /fætɪgə'bɪlətɪ/ n. 易疲劳性

serum /'sɪərəm/ n. 血清

calcium /'kælsɪəm/ n. 钙

malignancy /mə'lɪgnənsi/ n. 恶性(肿瘤等)

lipoprotein /'lɪpəprəʊtiːn/ n. 脂蛋白

specificity /ˌspesɪ'fɪsəti/ n. 特殊性

pivotal /'pɪvətl/ adj. 关键的

isotopic /aɪsəʊ'tɒpɪk/ adj. 同位素的

positron /'pɔzitrɔn/ n. 正电子

supplant /sə'plɑːnt/ v. 代替

vista /'vɪstə/ n. 展望

a battery of 一连串的

diagnosis. Nonetheless, patients must endure each of these tests, and the added cost of unnecessary testing is substantial. Furthermore, investigation of an unexpected abnormal finding may be associated with risk and/or expense and may lead to the diagnosis of an irrelevant or incidental problem. A skilled physician must learn to use these powerful diagnostic tools **judiciously**, always considering whether the results will alter management and benefit the patient. (928 words)

judiciously /dʒʊ'dɪʃəslɪ/
adv. 明智而审慎地

Notes:

1. Mendelian disorder: 孟德尔疾病，一种按孟德尔遗传形式出现的遗传性疾病。由 DNA 中单个突变引起，导致有某种或某些病理后果的单个基本缺陷，又称 monogenic (single-gene) disorder。
2. hyperparathyroidism: 甲状旁腺功能亢进，是指甲状旁腺分泌过多甲状旁腺激素 (PTH) 。甲状旁腺自身发生了病变，如过度增生、瘤性变甚至癌变，由于身体存在其他病症，如长期维生素 D 缺乏等都可能导致甲状旁腺功能亢进。甲状旁腺功能亢进可导致骨痛、骨折、高钙血症等，还可危害身体的其他多个系统，需积极诊治。
3. ultrasonography: 超声波检查法，是利用超声产生的波在人体内传播时，通过示波屏显示体内各种器官和组织对超声的反射和减弱规律来诊断疾病的一种方法。
4. positron emission tomography: 正电子成像术，简称 PET，是目前脑成像技术中应用最多的方法之一。当含有微量的放射性同位素葡萄糖溶液进入血液被大脑吸收后，PET 能检测到这种溶液发射的正电子。

While You Read

Task: Text-related Presentation

Directions: Take turns to make a 1-min presentation on the following topics. Your presentation should be based on the text but not limited to the text. You are encouraged to present in a unique and creative way.

1) Talk about the factors worthy of a doctor's note during the process of history-taking. (Para. 2)

2) State the reasons for performing a thorough and methodical physical examination. (Para. 4)

3) Talk about the advantages and disadvantages of laboratory tests. (Para. 5)

4) Talk about the reasons why physicians generally request multiple tests. (Para. 6)

5) Talk about the judicious choice made by a skilled physician when faced with findings from improved image studies. (Para. 8)

After You Read

Task 1: Academic English Study

Directions: Read this section carefully and try to find more examples of long sentences from Text A and Text B.

Complexity (II)

Long Sentences

Academic English is grammatically more complex than general English. It has more long sentences, like attributive clauses, subject clauses, adverbial clauses, predictive clauses, "to" complement clauses and sequences of prepositional phrases.

a. Attributive Clauses

Ex: An informative history is more than an orderly listing of symptoms; by listening to patients and noting the way *in which* they describe their symptoms, physicians can gain valuable insight into the problem. (Para. 2, Text A)

b. Subject Clauses

Ex: Pedagogically, *what* is tragic about tending to the iPatient is that it can't begin to compare with the joy, excitement, intellectual pleasure, pride, disappointment, and lessons in humility that trainees might experience by learning from the real patient's body examined at the bedside. (Para. 6, Text B)

c. Adverbial Clauses

Ex: Often, emergency room personnel have already scanned, tested, and diagnosed, *so that* interns meet a fully formed iPatient long before seeing the real patient. (Para. 4, Text B)

d. Predictive Clauses

Ex: Pedagogically, what is tragic about tending to the iPatient is *that* it can't begin to compare with the joy, excitement, intellectual pleasure, pride, disappointment. (Para. 6, Text B)

e. "to" Complement Clauses

Ex: The process of history-taking provides an opportunity *to* observe the patient's behavior and watch for features *to* be pursued more thoroughly during the physical examination. (Para. 2, Text A)

Task 2: Critical Thinking

Directions: Work in groups and discuss the following question. At the end of your discussion, each group will assign a representative to present your opinions on this issue.

With the help of the emerging hi-tech machines, doctors can make medical diagnosis much more easily. It turns out doctors, instead of examining the patients themselves, are asking patients to receive many tests which may be or may not be necessary. As a consequence, their clinical skills are in decline. Patients also tend to have more faith in the machinery diagnosis. What are the advantages and disadvantages of doctors' physical examination and that of machines? Can machines take the place of doctors in the future in terms of physical examination?

Text B

Before You Read

Task 1: Vocabulary Preview

Directions: Preview the words in the table below and use them to describe the following pictures.

endocarditis neurofibroma angioma tuning fork ophthalmoscope stethoscope

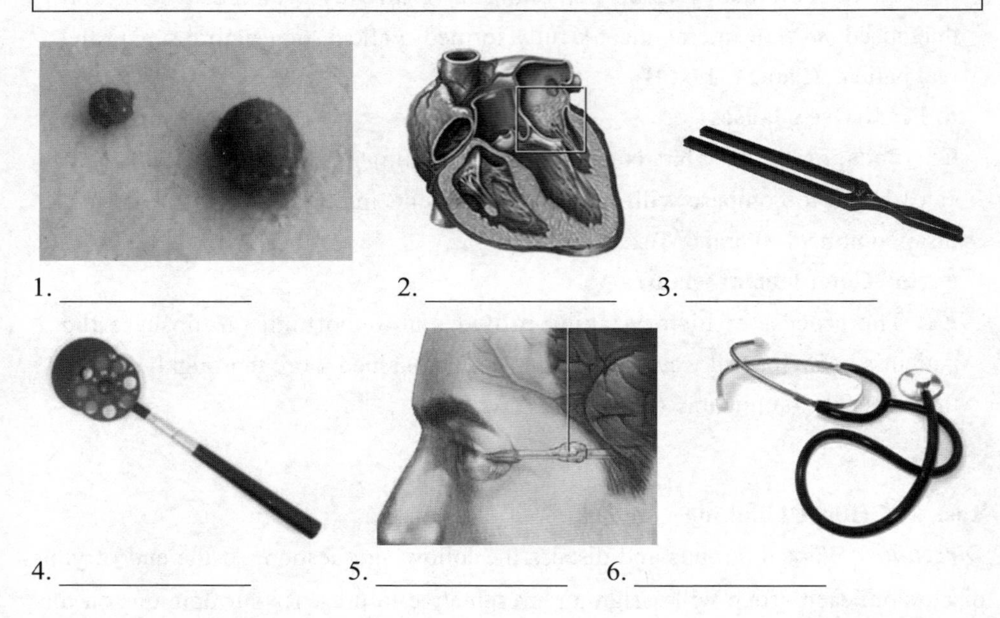

1. ____________ 2. ____________ 3. ____________

4. ____________ 5. ____________ 6. ____________

Task 2: Warming-up

Directions: Watch the video *Physician Qualifications* carefully and try to answer the questions below. While watching the video, please take notes in the blanks to help you follow the content.

1) What process should a future physician go through after graduating from college?

2) What majors do most people choose in their undergraduate years? And why?

3) Why does the speaker say the second two years in a medical school is more clinical?

4) What kind of personality is needed to be a good physician?

Notes

Text B Culture Shock — Patient as Icon, Icon as Patient

Abraham Verghese, M.D.

1. On my first day as an attending physician in a new hospital, I found my house staff and students in the team room, a **snug bunker** filled with glowing monitors[1]. Instead of sitting down to hear about the patients, I suggested we head out to see them. My team came willingly, though they probably felt that everything I would need to get up to speed[2] on our patients — the necessary images, the laboratory results — was right there in the team room. From my perspective, the most crucial element wasn't.

snug /snʌg/ adj. 舒适的

bunker /ˈbʌŋkə(r)/ n. 沙坑，燃料库

2. For the next few weeks, I ensured that we spent as little time as possible in the bunker. These were excellent residents who cared enormously about patients' welfare. They enjoyed being shown common findings — white nails of liver disease, an accessory nipple, **parotid** enlargement, spider **angiomas**, the **paradoxical** splitting of the second heart sound in left bundle branch block. Still, the demands of charting in the electronic medical record (EMR), moving patients through the system, and respecting work-hour limits led residents to spend an astonishing amount of time in front of the monitor; the EMR was their portal to consultative teams, the pharmacy, the laboratory, and radiology. It was meant

parotid /pəˈrɒtɪd/ adj. 腮腺的

angiomas /ˌændʒiˈəuməz/ n. 血管瘤

paradoxical /ˌpærəˈdɒksɪkl/ adj. 矛盾的

to serve them, but at times the opposite seemed true.

3. This ward experience highlighted for me an evolving tension between two approaches to patients. In the first way — call it the traditional way — the body is the text, a text that is changing and must be frequently inspected, **palpated**, **percussed**, and **auscultated**. The scent in the room, a family member's statement contradicting what the patient says, the **knobby** liver, **clonus**, the absent **nasolabial** fold, the hoarse voice — a multitude of such soundings help us understand the patient, and on this foundation, data from the chart can be selectively applied.

palpate /pælˈpeɪt/ v. 触诊
percuss /pɜːˈkʌs/ v. 轻敲
auscultate /ˈɔːskəlteɪt/ v. 听诊
knobby /ˈnɒbɪ/ adj. 多节的
clonus /ˈkləʊnəs/ n. 阵挛，抽筋
nasolabial /neɪˈsəʊleɪbɪəl/ adj. 鼻唇的

4. The other way — call it the **expedient** way — is not formally taught, and yet residents seem to have learned it no matter where in the United States they trained. The patient is still at the center, but more as an icon for another entity clothed in binary garments[3]: the "iPatient."Often, emergency room personnel have already scanned, tested, and diagnosed, so that interns meet a fully formed iPatient long before seeing the real patient. The iPatient's blood counts and **emanations** are tracked and trended like a Dow Jones Index, and **pop-up** flags[4] remind caregivers to feed or bleed. iPatients are handily discussed (or "card-flipped") in the bunker, while the real patients keep the beds warm and ensure that the folders bearing their names stay alive on the computer.

expedient /ɪkˈspiːdiənt/ adj. 方便的
emanation /ˌeməˈneɪʃn/ n. 发出，散发
pop-up /ˈpɔpˌʌp/ adj. 弹起的

5. If one **eschews** the skilled and repeated examination of the real patient, then simple diagnoses and new developments are overlooked, while tests, consultations, and procedures that might not be needed are ordered. Every seasoned attending physician has seen examples of this error mode: **distended** neck veins, weight gain, and **cardiomegaly** labeled as pneumonia instead of **congestive** heart failure because the infiltrates on a chest x-ray were given too much weight; missed **embolic lesions** of **endocarditis** in a **febrile** patient; a report by the intern of "small **intra-abdominal** masses" that were in fact **subcutaneous neurofibromas** also abundant on chest, forearms, thighs—anywhere an examiner might lay a hand. The financial costs of imprecise observations that lead to unnecessary or risky investigations are not known; in a health care system in which our menu has no prices, we can order filet mignon at every meal.

eschew /ɪs'tʃuː/ v. 避开
distend /dɪ'stend/ vt. 使……膨胀
cadiomegaly /kɑːdɪəʊ'megəlɪ/ n. 心脏扩大症
congestive /kən'dʒestɪv/ adj. 充血的
embolic /em'bɒlɪk/ adj. 插子的
lesion /'liːʒn/ n. 损害
endocarditis /ˌendəʊkɑː'daɪtɪs/ n. 心内膜炎
febrile /'fiːbraɪl/ adj. 发热的
intra-abdominal/'ɪntrəæbd'ɒmɪnl/ adj. 腹内的
subcutaneous /ˌsʌbkju'teɪniəs/ adj. 皮下的
neurofibroma/ˌnjʊərəʊfaɪ'brəʊmə/ n. 纤维神经瘤

6. **Pedagogically**, what is tragic about tending to the iPatient is that it can't begin to compare with the joy, excitement, intellectual pleasure, pride, disappointment, and lessons in humility that trainees might experience by learning from the real patient's body examined at the bedside. When residents don't witness the bedside-**sleuth** aspect of our discipline—its underlying romance and passion—they may come to view internal medicine as a trade practiced before a computer screen.

pedagogically /ˌpedə'gɒdʒɪklɪ/ adv. 教学法上
sleuth /sluːθ/ n. 侦探

7. If we in academia have managed to ignore the loss of bedside skills, our patients see the deficiency easily. Patients recognize how the **perfunctory** bedside visit, the **stethoscope** placement, through clothing, on the **sternum** like the blessing of a **potentate**'s **scepter**[5], differs from a skilled, hands-on exam. Rituals are about transformation, and when performed well, this ritual, at a minimum, suggests attentiveness and inspires confidence in the physician.

perfunctory /pə'fʌŋktəri/ adj. 敷衍的
stethoscope /'steθəskəʊp/ n. 听诊器
sternum /'stɜːnəm/ n. 胸骨
potentate /'stɜːnəm/ n. 统治者
scepter /'septə/ n. 节杖（象征君权）

8. In my years of teaching, I've found that residents increasingly approach the patient with little expectation of discovering tangible findings. When such a finding presents itself, it is the exceptional resident who pursues and refines the observation, most being content to murmur vaguely about a murmur[6] without describing its qualities, the presence of a **parasternal** heave, or key **ancillary** findings. Because the echocardiogram, magnetic resonance image (MRI), and computed tomographic scan precisely characterize anatomy, the physical exam is too often viewed as redundant. Indeed, the EMR template requires just one click to fill in, "Heart: regular rate and rhythm, no murmurs," and it is an effort to change it. In short, bedside skills have deteriorated as the available technology has evolved.

parasternal /pæ'rəstɜːnl/ adj. 胸骨旁的
ancillary /æn'sɪlərɪ/ adj. 辅助的

9. How did we reach this state of affairs? The fault is ours as teachers of medicine.

We don't expect much from trainees at the bedside. If we did, we'd insist they carry **ophthalmoscopes**, **tuning forks**, and tendon hammers. Being the attending on a teaching service nowadays requires visiting once or twice daily, being present for procedures, and documenting everything. Senior physicians with strong bedside skills are opting out of[7] this time-consuming duty, so residents have little exposure to them. Attendings are therefore often recently trained internists, knowledgeable about hospital—based systems, quality measures, critical pathways, and **informatics** — but the bedside exam may not be an area of interest or strength.

ophthalmoscope /ɒf'θælmə,skəʊp/ n. 检眼镜；眼底镜

tuning forks 音叉

informatics /ˌɪnfə'mætɪks/ n. 信息学

10. I feel fortunate to live in this age of incredible technology, with its remarkable new ways of seeing the body. I am excited about portable ultrasonography, for example, which allows us to instantly confirm findings at the bedside and discover the limits of our own skills. We need more of that kind of translational work — to develop the next generation of stethoscopes, ophthalmoscopes, and tendon hammers. Surely having physicians become more **discerning**, more comfortable, and eager to spend more time at the bedside is a good thing for patients. For the clinician, the bedside is **hallowed** ground, the place where fellow human beings allow us the privilege of looking at, touching, and listening to their bodies. Our skills and discernment must be worthy of such trust. (1076 words)

discerning /dɪ'sɜːnɪŋ/ adj. 有辨识能力的

hallowed /'hæləʊd/ adj. 神圣的

Notes:

1. a snug bunker filled with glowing monitors: 放满发光发热的监测仪的、建造良好的燃料库，形容前文的 team room 里到处都是在工作着的监测仪，设备齐全且精良。
2. get up to speed: 熟悉了解新项目的详细情况
3. as an icon for another entity clothed in binary garments: 作为另一个穿着二进制衣服的实体的标志，表示病人的几乎一切体征都先通过仪器检测，而不是传统方式的医生亲自检查，变成了 iPatient。
4. pop-up flags: 系统突然弹出来的提示
5. like the blessing of a potentate's scepter: 就像受到了皇上的宠幸一般，此处暗指病人可以看出医生检查的敷衍，连在胸骨上放置听诊器都像是一种特殊的优待。a potentate's scepter 原指统治者的节杖，象征着君权。
6. murmur vaguely about a murmur: 含糊不清地低声咕哝着某个心脏杂音，前一个 murmur 意为低声咕哝，后一个 murmur 指心脏杂音。
7. opt out of: 决定不参加……

While You Read

Task 1: Reading Skills

Directions: As is mentioned in the ***Skills Bank***, students can recognize relationships within sentences through addition, clarification, comparison, contrast, example, location or spatial order, cause and effect, summary, and time. Try to find at least one sentence from Text B to illustrate each way above.

Ways to recognize relationships within sentences	Sentence to illustrate
Addition	*Being the attending on a teaching service nowadays requires visiting once or twice daily, being present for procedures, and documenting everything.*
Clarification	
Comparison	
Contrast	

续表

Ways to recognize relationships within sentences	Sentence to illustrate
Example	
Location and spatial order	
Cause and effect	
Summary	
Time	

Task 2: Text-related Presentation

Directions: Take turns to make a 1-min presentation on the following topics. Your presentation should be based on the text but not limited to the text. You are encouraged to present in a unique and creative way.

1) Introduce the concept of electronic medical record (EMR). (Para. 2)
2) Draw a comparison between the two approaches to patients. (Para. 3-Para.4)
3) Talk about the potential problems of tending to the iPatient. (Para. 5)
4) Compare the different experiences patients get from a skilled hands-on exam and perfunctory bedside visit. (Para. 7)
5) Analyze the reasons for doctors' deteriorating bedside skills. (Para. 8-Para.9)

After You Read

Task 1: Oral Presenting

Directions: Try to rephrase or explain the following sentences without using the boldfaced words or phrases.(This is going to be integrated into the communicative interaction in the classroom. The task can be done orally in the classroom.)

1. The EMR **was meant to** serve them, but **at times the opposite** seemed true.
2. Often, emergency room personnel have already scanned, tested, and diagnosed, so that interns meet **a fully formed** iPatient **long before** seeing the real patient.
3. In my years of teaching, I've found that residents **increasingly approach** the

patient **with little expectation of** discovering **tangible findings**.

4. Senior physicians with strong bedside skills **are opting out of** this **time-consuming duty**, so residents **have little exposure to** them.
5. I feel fortunate to live **in this age of** incredible technology, with **its remarkable new ways** of seeing the body.

Task 2: Critical Thinking

Directions: Work in groups and discuss the following questions. At the end of your discussion, each group will assign a representative to present your points on this issue.

1) What's the ideal relationship between a physician and a patient?

2) What kind of problems will iPatients have?

3) What should teachers of medicine do to reverse the state of deteriorating bedside skills?

After-class Tasks

Task 1: Word Chunks

Directions: Complete the following word chunks taken from Text A and Text B according to their Chinese equivalents and make a sentence with each word chunk.

1. ________ the patient ________ 让病人放松
2. be performed ________ 系统性地操作
3. from ________ to ________ 从头到脚
4. skill in ________ 物理诊断技能
5. ________ tests 高灵敏度的诊断性测试
6. ________ tests 实验室测试
7. abnormalities of ________ 肝功能失常
8. ________ cholesterol 低浓度脂蛋白胆固醇
9. a ________ factor 关键因素
10. ________ 住院医师
11. electronic ________ 电子病历
12. the ________ way 方便的方式
13. ________ attending physicians 有经验的主治医师
14. ________ confidence 激发信心
15. the ________ resident 杰出的住院医师
16. ________ of 决定不参加
17. ________ duty 耗时的责任
18. an area ________ 感兴趣的领域
19. discover ________ of 发现……的限制
20. ________ work 转化工作

Task 2: Translation

Directions: Translate sentence 1 to 3 into Chinese and pay close attention to the translation of the words in bold. Then translate sentence 4 to 6 into English using the words in the bracket.

1. The patient should **have the opportunity to** tell his or her own story of the illness **without frequent interruption** and receive **expressions of** interest, encouragement, and empathy from the physician.

___

___

2. Because patients **vary** in their medical sophistication and ability to recall facts, the reported medical history should **be corroborated whenever possible**.

___

___

3. If one **eschews** the **skilled and repeated examination** of the real patient, then simple diagnoses and new developments **are overlooked**, while tests, consultations, and procedures that might not be needed are ordered.

___

___

4. 通常，只有当病人与医生相处融洽时，他们才会提供完整的信息。因此让病人在最大程度上放松有助于医生获取足够的病史资料。(put ... at ease)

___

___

5. 因为有许多高灵敏度的诊断测试的存在，特别是成像技术，人们对体格检查的重视度变得越来越低。(put emphasis on)

___

___

6. 我的团队成员可能觉得我尽快了解病人病情所需要的资料，如片子和检查结果，都一一摆在那里。(get up to speed)

___

___

Task 3: Listening & Speaking

Directions: Listen to the tape and finish the guided note-taking.

Word Bank

buck the trend 反潮流
orthopedic /ɔːθəʊ'piːdɪk/ adj. 整形手术的
rabbi /'ræbaɪ/ n. 犹太教士
heart valve 心脏瓣膜
ankle reflex 踝反射
disrobe /dɪs'rəʊb/ v. 脱去衣服

Dr. Wasfy thinks that doctors are now often doing expensive tests where, in the past, 1) ________ would have given the same information.

Dr. Roman Desanctis points out that this is not 2) ________ when he saw apatient whose lungs were 3) ________, but his primary care doctor had totally missed it.

Many doctors have abandoned the physical exam. But some are bucking the trend. Dr. Basgoz and Dr. Verghese are among the latter group of doctors.

Dr. Basgoz:

She says many young doctors don't understand why they should bother to 4) ________.
She says she is definitely worried that the physical exam 5) ________.

Dr. Verghese:

He blames much of the trend on American doctors' 6) ________.
He believes that doctors often spend so much time with that entity7) ________. He calls it the 8) ________, like iPad and your iPhone.
His worst nightmare is that someone passes through his hands with a 9) ________, treatable condition because of 10) ________.

Task 4: Research

Directions: When you need to see a doctor, will you choose a general practitioner or a specialist? Do some research into *the differences between general practice and internal medicine*, and then brainstorm the following aspects in groups before developing your discussions into an oral presentation for the next class. You can present in the form of an interview, short play or simply a lecture. Make sure each member of the group will present his or her part on the stage.

1) The definition of general practice
2) The definition of internal medicine
3) The responsibilities of GP
4) The responsibilities of internists

5) Education and training
6) Difference in the treatment provided

Resources

Here are some websites where you can find useful information for your research.
http://www.ehow.com/about_6555489_difference-general-practitioner-internal-medicine_.html
http://www.differencebetween.net/science/health/difference-between-general-practice-and-internal-medicine/
http://www.merchantcircle.com/articles/Doctor-of-Internal-Medicine-VS-General-Practitioners/1002759

Task 5: Writing

Directions: In the United States, physician candidates must complete eight years of medical school before becoming a qualified physician. They should receive classroom instruction in life sciences and fundamentals ofmedicalcare. After that, they need to explore the nature of a physician's work through a series of practical rotations in hospitals or other healthcare facilities. Upon completion of an M.D. program, candidates embark upon one-to-three years of paid residency training.

Is it worthwhile to devote such a long time to the preparation for a career? Please write an essay on the topic ***My View on Becoming a Physician***.

Task6: Vocabulary Log

Directions: Please finish the vocabulary log (Please find the log at the end of the book) by looking up the dictionary and write down the words or expressions you have learnt in this unit by following the examples already listed in the log. And then write down the translation for each vocabulary item and if possible, its variants, synonym, antonym and the frequent collocations.

Task 7: Reading Log

Directions: After learning the whole unit and conducting the research, you have known more about physicians from different perspectives. You can go to the library or surf on the internet for more knowledge about it. You can take down the key information according to the sample chart. (Please find the chart at the end of the book) Also you are allowed to complete the chart on a computer or tablet so that this section is expandable if you want to write more than the space on a paper form might allow. And then send it to your teacher by emails. The reading log can serve as an informal way to keep track of your reading progress.

Unit 5

Birth of Modern Surgery

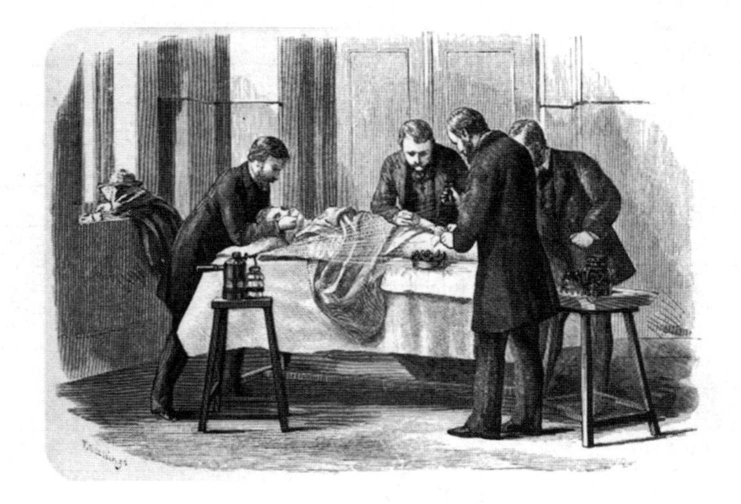

We ought to have saints' days to commemorate the great discoveries which have been made for all mankind, and perhaps for all time. Nature is a prodigal of pain. I should like to find a day when we can take a holiday, a day of jubilation when we can fête good Saint Anesthesia and chaste and pure Saint Antiseptic.

——Winston Churchill

Pre-class Tasks

Task 1: Medical Terminology Study

Directions: Study the word roots, prefixes and suffixes listed in the table below and do the **Vocabulary Preview** exercise for Text A or / and Text B according to your teacher's instructions.

Roots	**Meaning**
mort/o	death 死亡
arter/o, arteri/o	artery 动脉
aneurysm/o	aneurysm 动脉瘤
an/o	anus 肛门
fistul/o	fistula 瘘
herni/o	hernia 疝
col/o, colon/o,	colon 结肠
ile/o	ileum 回肠
seps/o	infection 感染，传
arthr/o	joint 关节
path/o	disease 疾病
hem/o	blood 血
Prefixes	**Meaning**
intra-	within 在内，内，内部
anti-	against 反，对抗，解，抑制，退，代替
Suffixes	**Meaning**
-stomy	creation of an opening 造口术，吻合术
-sepsis	putrefaction 腐坏，腐败
-itis	inflammation 炎
-logy	study of ……学
-rrhage	burst forth 出血，流血
-stasis	stopping, standing 固定，停滞，郁滞

Task 2: Prepared Individual Presentation

Directions: The assigned students need to prepare a 1-min oral presentation concerning the questions in **Text-related Presentation** for Text A and/or Text B as required by your teacher.

Task 3: The Muddiest Points

Directions:Read Text A and Text B in the study group to find out the sentences that are the least clear to you after your discussions, the viewpoints that you disagree with and the understanding you have achieved through discussions and the questions you want to put forward concerning the content of the texts. Put the above information in a slip and send it to the teacher via WeChat 24 hours prior to the class. (The slip can be found on the last page of the book.)

Skills Bank

Distinguishing Facts and Opinions

Generally speaking, a fact is something that has actually happened or that is empirically true and can be supported by evidence. An opinion is a belief; it is normally subjective, meaning that it can vary based on a person's perspective, emotions, or individual understanding of something. For example, biological differences between males and females are a fact, while a preference for one gender over the other is opinion.

According to most definitions, something is a fact if it matches objective reality. For something to be objective, it must be outside of the mind and not be based on feelings or biases. This is the opposite of an opinion, which is what an individual thinks or feels about a subject.

Facts

There are two important details you must know about facts.

1. A fact can be either a true or a false statement.
2. A fact can be proven true or false through observation or data collection.

Opinions

It is very important to know the following characteristics of statements of opinion.

1. Any statement that expresses the possibility or probability of an event that CANNOT be proven true or false through observation or data collection is an OPINION.
2. Any statement that concerns the future or future events is a statement of OPINION. This is true even if the statements seem probable. No one can know the future objectively; therefore, future statements are statements of opinion.

In-class Tasks

Text A

Before You Read

Task 1: Vocabulary Preview

Directions: Divide the following words into their word parts and then give their Chinese translations based on the table above.

Medical Terms	Prefix	Word Root(s)	Suffix	Chinese
mortality				
artery				
anal				
fistula				
colostomy				
ileostomy				
intradermal				
antisepsis				
arthritis				
pathology				
hemorrhage				
hemostasis				

Task 2: Warming-up

Directions: Watch the video carefully and try to answer the questions below. While watching the video, please take some notes in the blanks to help you to memorize the information.

1) What is surgery about and what do surgeons do according to your understanding?

2) According to the video, what was surgery like in ancient times?

3) Who and what promoted the development of modern surgery?

4) What else do you think play important roles in the birth of modern surgery?

Notes

Text A Historical Relationship Between Medicine and Surgery

1. Despite outward appearances, it was actually not until the latter decades of the 19th century that the surgeon truly emerged as a specialist within the whole **arena** of medicine to become a recognized and respected clinical physician. Similarly, it was not until the first decades of the 20th century that surgery could be considered to have achieved the status of a bona fide[1] profession. Before this time, the scope of surgery remained limited. Surgeons, or at least those medical men who used the **sobriquet** surgeon, whether university-educated or trained in private **apprenticeships**, at best treated only simple **fractures**, **dislocations**, and **abscesses** and occasionally performed **amputations** with dexterity[2], but also with high mortality rates[3]. They managed to **ligate** major arteries for common and accessible **aneurysms** and made heroic attempts to excise external tumors. Some individuals focused on the treatment

arena /ə'riːnə/ n. 竞技场

sobriquet /'səʊbrɪkeɪ/ n. 绰号

apprenticeship /ə'prentɪʃɪp/ n. 学徒期

fracture /'fræktʃə(r)/ n. 骨折

dislocation /ˌdɪslə'keɪʃn/ n. 脱臼

abscess /'æbses/ n. 脓肿

amputation /ˌæmpjʊ'teɪʃn/ n. 截肢术

ligate /lɪ'geɪt/ v. 结扎，绑

aneurysm /'ænjərɪzəm/ n. 动脉瘤

of anal fistulas[4], **hernias**, **cataracts**, and bladder stones[5]. **Inept** attempts at reduction of incarcerated[6] and strangulated[7] hernias were made and, hesitatingly, rather **rudimentary** colostomies or ileostomies[8] were created by simply incising the skin over an expanding **intra-abdominal** mass, which represented the end stage of a long-standing intestinal obstruction[9]. Compound fractures of the limbs, with attendant sepsis, remained mostly unmanageable, with **staggering** morbidity being a likely surgical outcome. Although a few bold surgeons endeavored to incise the abdomen in the hope of dividing obstructing bands and **adhesions**, abdominal and other types of intrabody surgery were almost unknown.

hernia/ˈhɜːnɪə/ n. 疝
cataract /ˈkætərækt/ n. 白内障
inept /ɪˈnept/ adj. 不熟练的
rudimentary /ˌruːdɪˈmentri/ adj. 基本的
incise /ɪnˈsaɪz/ v. 切，切开
intra-abdominal /ˈɪntrəæbdˈɒmɪnl/ adj. 腹内的
staggering /ˈstægərɪŋ/adj. 令人震惊的
adhesion /ədˈhiːʒn/ n. 粘连

2. Despite it all, including an ignorance of anesthesia and **antisepsis** tempered with[10] the not uncommon result of the patient suffering from or succumbing to[11] the effects of a surgical operation (or both), surgery was long considered an important and medically valid therapy. This seeming paradox, in view of the terrifying nature of surgical intervention, its limited technical scope, and its **damning** consequences before the development of modern conditions, is explained by the simple fact that surgical procedures were usually performed only for external difficulties that required an objective anatomic diagnosis[12]. Surgeons or followers of the surgical cause saw what needed to be fixed (e.g., abscesses, broken bones, **bulging** tumors, cataracts, hernias)

antisepsis /ˌæntɪˈsepsɪs/ n. 防腐，消毒
damning /ˈdæmɪŋ/ adj. 毁灭的
bulging /ˈbʌldʒɪŋ/ adj. 鼓起的

and would treat the problem in as rational a manner as the times permitted. **Conversely**, the physician was forced to **render** subjective care for disease processes that were neither visible nor understood. After all, it is a difficult task to treat the symptoms of illnesses such as arthritis, asthma, heart failure, and diabetes, to name but a few, if there is no scientific understanding or internal knowledge of what **constitutes** their basic pathologic and physiologic **underpinnings**.

conversely /'kɒnvɜːsli/ adv. 相反地

render /'rendə(r)/ v. 给予

constitute /'kɒnstɪtjuːt/ v. 组成，构成

underpinning /'ʌndəˌpiniŋ/ n. 基础

3. With the breathtaking advances made in pathologic anatomy[13] and experimental physiology[14] during the 18th and first part of the 19th centuries, physicians would soon adopt a therapeutic viewpoint that had long been prevalent among surgeons. It was no longer a question of just treating symptoms; the actual pathologic problem could ultimately be understood. Internal disease processes that manifested themselves through difficult-to-treat external signs and symptoms were finally described via physiology-based experimentation or viewed pathologically through the lens of a microscope. Because this **reorientation** of internal medicine occurred within a relatively short time and brought about such dramatic results in the classification, diagnosis, and treatment of disease, the rapid **ascent** of mid-19th century internal medicine might seem more impressive than the agonizingly slow, but steady, advance of surgery. In a seeming contradiction of mid-19th

reorientation /ˌriːɔːrɪən'teɪʃn/ n. 再定位

ascent /ə'sent/ n. 上升；升高

century scientific and social reality, medicine appeared as the more progressive branch, with surgery lagging behind. The art and craft of surgery, for all its practical possibilities, would be severely restricted until the discovery of anesthesia in 1846 and an understanding and acceptance of the need for surgical antisepsis and asepsis during the 1870s and 1880s. Still, surgeons never needed a diagnostic and pathologic revolution in the manner of the physician. Despite the imperfection of their scientific knowledge, the pre–modern era surgeon did cure with some technical confidence.

4. That the gradual evolution of surgery was **superseded** in the 1880s and 1890s by the rapid introduction of startling new technical advances was based on a simple **culminating axiom**—the four fundamental clinical **prerequisites** that were required before a surgical operation could ever be considered a truly **viable** therapeutic procedure had finally been identified and understood:

1) Knowledge of human anatomy

2) Method of controlling **hemorrhage** and maintaining intraoperative **hemostasis**

3) Anesthesia to permit the performance of pain-free procedures

4) Explanation of the nature of infection, along with the elaboration of methods necessary to achieve an antiseptic and aseptic operating room environment

supersede /ˌsuːpəˈsiːd/ v. 代替

culminating /kʌlˈmɪneɪtɪŋ/ adj. 终极的

axiom /ˈæksiəm/ n. 公理

prerequisite /ˌpriːˈrekwəzɪt/ n. 前提

viable /ˈvaɪəbl/ adj. 切实可行的

hemorrhage /ˈhemərɪdʒ/ n. 大出血

hemostasis/ˌhiːməˈsteɪsɪs/ n. 止血

5. The first two prerequisites were essentially solved in the 16th century, but the latter two would not be fully resolved until the ending decades of the 19th century. In turn, the ascent of 20th century scientific surgery would unify the profession and allow what had always been an art and craft to become a learned vocation. Standardized postgraduate surgical education and training programs could be established to help produce a cadre of[15] scientifically knowledgeable physicians. Moreover, in a final **snub** to an unscientific past, newly established basic surgical research laboratories offered the means of proving or disproving the latest theories while providing a testing ground for bold and exciting clinical breakthroughs. (863 words)

snub /snʌb/ n. 冷落，怠慢

Notes:

1. bona fide: 真实的，真诚的
2. with dexterity: 尤其是指外科手术的时候，医生手法灵活
3. mortality rate: 死亡率
4. anal fistula: 肛瘘
5. bladder stone: 膀胱结石
6. incarcerated hernias: 箝闭性疝
7. strangulated hernias: 绞窄性疝
8. colostomies or ileostomy: 结肠造口术或者回肠造口术
9. intestinal obstruction: 肠梗阻
10. temper with: 调和或减轻某事物的作用
11. succumb to: 感染或者死于（某种疾病）
12. anatomic diagnosis: 定位诊断
13. pathologic anatomy: 病理解剖学
14. experimental physiology : 实验生理学
15. a cadre of : 一批（人）

While You Read

Task: Text-related Presentation

Directions: Take turns to make a 1-min presentation about the following topics. Your presentation should be based on the text but not limited to the text. You are encouraged to present in a unique and creative way.

1) Talk about the role and position of surgeons before the 19th century. (Para.1)

2) Give us a brief introduction about surgery and internal medicine in the 19th century. (Para.2)

3) Talk about pathologic anatomy in the first part of 19th century and surgical development in that period. (Para.3)

4) What is therapeutic viewpoint of physicians? (Para.3)

5) Explain your understanding of "the art and craft of surgery" based on the text. (Para.3)

After You Read

Task 1: Academic English Study

Directions: Read this section carefully and try to find more examples of lexical density and complexity as shown below from Text A and Text B.

Complexity (III)

Lexical Density & Complexity

Academic language is relatively more complex in that it has higher lexical density and complexity.

Lexical density

If we define lexical density as the number of content words in a clause, then academic English has a higher lexical density than general English.

Ex: Despite it all, including an ignorance of anesthesia and antisepsis tempered with the not uncommon result of the patient suffering from or succumbing to the effects of a surgical operation (or both), surgery was long considered an important and medically valid therapy. (Para.2)

Lexical complexity

Adding affixes to existing words (the base) to form new words is common in academic English. Prefixes are added to the front of the base (like dislike), whereas suffixes are added to the end of the base (active activate). Prefixes usually do not change the class of the base word, but suffixes usually do change the class of the word.

The most common prefixes used to form new verbs in academic English are: re-, dis-, over-, un-, mis-, out-. The most common suffixes are: -ise, -en, -ate, -(i)fy. By far the most common affix in academic English is -ise.

Task 2: Critical Thinking

Directions: Work in groups and discuss the following questions. At the end of your discussion, each group will assign a representative to present your opinions on this issue.

Henry Sigerist, widely regarded as the greatest medical historian in the 20th century, once said "Surgery became great, not because anesthesia and antisepsis were introduced, but anesthesia and antisepsis were found because surgery was to become great". The observation seems to attribute the advancement of surgery to the matrix of social trends that facilitate individuals to pursue safer and better technologies in surgery. Is the process inevitable? What's your view on the relationship between individual achievement and social progress? Use specific examples to support your arguments.

Text B

Before You Read

Task 1: Vocabulary Preview

Directions: Preview the words in the table below and use them to describe the following pictures.

cataract	antiseptic	suppuration
tissue	fracture	germ

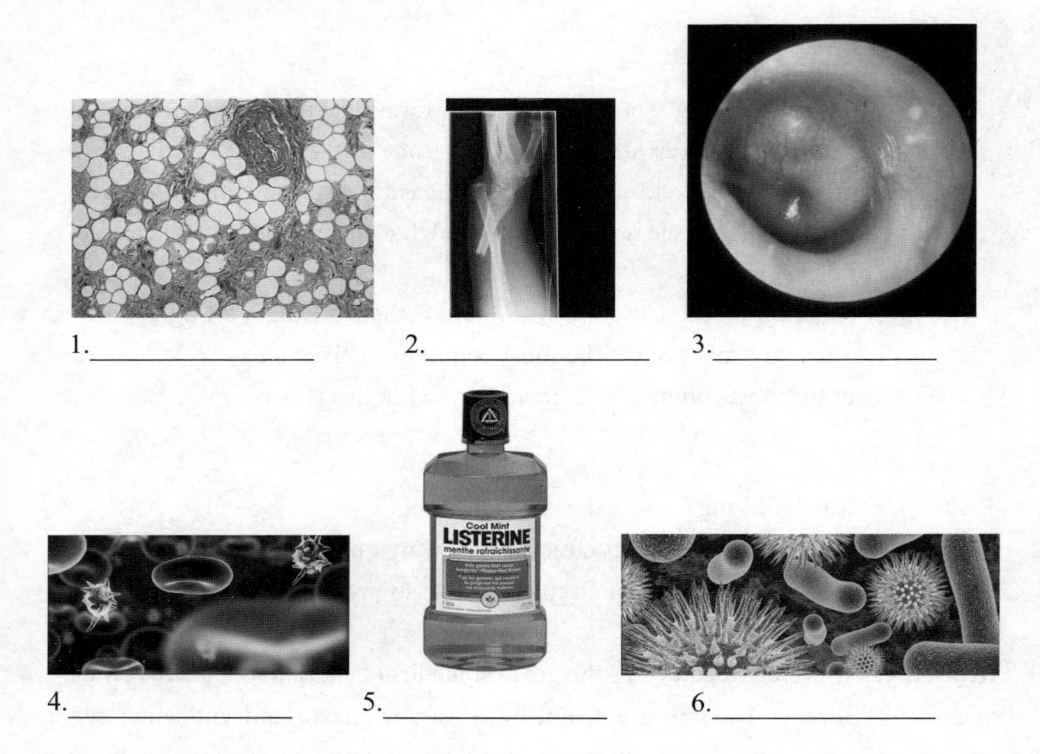

1.________ 2.________ 3.________

4.________ 5.________ 6.________

Task 2: Warming-up

Directions: Watch the video carefully and try to answer the questions below. While watching the video, please take some notes in the blanks to help you to memorize the information.

1) Who was the video talking about?

2) What contributions did the man make in the field of modern surgery according to the video?

Notes

Text B Joseph Lister: Father of Modern Surgery

1. On the **centenary** of Joseph Lister's death, it is appropriate to remember and honor his remarkable accomplishments that earned him the title"father of modern surgery".

centenary /sen'tiːnəri/ n. 一百年纪念

2. It was Lister's genius to take the work of Pasteur on the **etiology** of **fermentation** and envision this process as the same that was causing infection and **gangrene**. In the face of movements to abolish all surgery in hospitals because of the prohibitive death rate from infection, Lister changed the treatment of compound fractures[1] from **amputation** to limb preservation and opened the way for abdominal and other intra-cavity surgery.

etiology /ˌiːtɪ'ɒlədʒɪ/ n. 病因学
fermentation /ˌfɜːmen'teɪʃn/ n. 发酵
gangrene /'gæŋgriːn/ n. 坏疽
amputation /ˌæmpjʊ'teɪʃn/ n. 截肢

3. Born in Essex, England, to a Quaker family[2], his father was elected a Fellow of the Royal Society for his construction of the first **achromatic** lens and coauthored a paper with Thomas Hodgkin[3] about red blood cells. Paternal guidance was a major influence throughout Lister's career.

achromatic /ˌækrəʊ'mætɪk/ adj. 消色差的

4. Lister was an excellent student at the University College of University of London and became house surgeon[4] at University College Hospital where he attained Fellowship in the Royal College of Surgeons. On the advice of Professor Sharpely of physiology, he went to study under the renowned surgeon James Syme in Edinburgh. Lister prospered in Edinburgh and married Syme's eldest daughter, Agnes.

5. His main research interest was inflammation, a process then considered a specific disease and not a response by healthy tissues to infection. Lister did come to understand that inflammation caused loss of vitality, which rendered tissues helpless as if they were dead, helpless against organisms he would eventually attribute as the cause of the **devastating** and feared surgical site infections. He published 15 papers about the action of muscles in the skin and the eye, the **coagulation** of blood and blood vessel changes with infection.

devastating /ˈdevəsteɪtɪŋ/ adj. 毁灭性的，灾难性的

coagulation /kəʊˌægjʊˈleɪʃn/ n. 凝结，凝结物

6. At 33 years of age, he was appointed Regius Professor[5] of Surgery at the University of Glasgow, but it took him another year to get privileges at the Glasgow Royal **Infirmary**. His initial application was rejected by the Chair of the Royal Infirmary Board, David Smith, with the comment "But our institution is a curative one. It is not an educational one." Glasgow had twice the population of Edinburgh and was renowned for its "warmhearted, **voluble** and uncritically friendly inhabitants," an ideal environment for a young surgeon to embark on a new, unproven treatment regime.

infirmary/ɪnˈfɜːməri/ n. 医院

voluble /ˈvɒljʊbl/ adj. 爱说话的

7. The world of surgery when Lister began his practice was primitive by our standards. Although Fracastoro of Verona in 1546 **theorized** that small germs could cause **contagious** diseases, no one associated them with wound infections. Bed linen and laboratory coats were not washed and surgical

theorize /ˈθiəraiz/ v. 创建理论

contagious /kənˈteɪdʒəs/ adj. 传染性的

instruments were only cleaned before they were put away for storage. The same **probe** was used for the wounds of all patients during rounds to look for pockets of undrained pus[6]. **Suppuration** and laudable pus[7] were considered part of normal healing. Operative procedures were only occasionally performed in the average surgeon's practice,and there was talk of banning all surgery from hospitals because of **septic** complications. Sir J.E.Erichsen, a future President of the Royal College of Surgeons[8], stated "The abdomen, chest and brain will forever be closed to operations by a wise and humane surgeon."

probe /prəʊb/ n. 探针

suppuration /ˌsʌpjʊˈreɪʃn/ n. 脓

septic /ˈseptɪk/ adj. 感染的

8. Lister's interest in wound healing began when he worked as a dresser for Sir Erichsen. Erichsen believed the wounds were infected from **miasmas** that arose from the wound themselves and became concentrated in the air. Erichsen had deduced that more than 7 patients with an infected wound in a 14-bed ward led to **saturation** of the air and spread of the dangerous gasses causing gangrene. Lister was not convinced, as when the wounds were **debrided** and cleaned, some wounds healed. This sparked his suspicion that something in the wound itself was at fault.

miasmas /miˈæzmə/ n. 瘴气

saturation /ˌsætʃəˈreɪʃn/ n. 饱和状态

debride /dɪˈbraɪd/ v. 清除

9. Lister's great intellectual breakthrough came when, on the advice of Thomas Anderson, a Glasgow professor of chemistry, he read Pasteur's[9] papers, *Recherches sur la putrefaction*, and **postulated** that the same process causing fermentation was involved

postulate /ˈpɒstjuleɪt/ v. 假定

with wound sepsis. Having heard of **creosote** being used to disinfect sewage, he applied carbolic acid[10] compounds as an antiseptic on surgical wounds. Having observed the marked difference in morbidity and mortality between simple and compound fractures, he postulated that infection came from exposure to the air in compound fractures without the protection of the skin. He began his antiseptic method with compound fracture wounds because the standard treatment of amputation was always available should his method fail.The results of this new method of treating wounds were soon apparent,and it then did not "seem right to withhold it longer from the profession generally." His work was initially published in 2 papers in the *Lancet*[11]; the first in March 1867, the second in July of the same year.

creosote /ˈkriːəsəʊt/ n. 木馏油

10. Lister made many alterations to his method of wound care, and the **iconic** carbolic acid spray was only 1 part of the evolution of antisepsis. The **skepticism** and opposition from some of his colleagues is legendary, as was the enthusiasm when the positive results were evident in the patients. Germany led the way in adopting Lister's antiseptic technique, followed by the United States, France and lastly Great Britain. Some of this opposition was understandable, as germs were too small to be seen in their microscopes, and Lister thought the air was the sole source of **contamination**. He received **accolade**s and prestigious awards from many nations and was appointed a Peer [12]in Great Britain.

iconic /aɪˈkɒnɪk/ adj. 标志性的

skepticism /ˈskeptɪsɪzəm/ n. 怀疑态度

contamination /kənˌtæmɪˈneɪʃən/ n. 污染

accolade /ˈækəleɪd/ n. 嘉奖，表扬

11. Lister was only human, and history has duly recorded some imperfections. Although his students had the utmost respect and praise for him, **collegiality** in Glasgow was a problem, and he neglected to share credit for his success with other members of the Glasgow team, to the great **chagrin** of the Royal Infirmary administration. Harsh criticism of the system of medical teaching in London almost cost him his appointment to King's College Hospital at the peak of his career, and he failed to support equality of women with men in medicine. Although **asepsis** and **sterile** technique have replaced antisepsis as the primary principle in combating infection, it was Lister's application of germ theory to the care of surgical patients that laid the foundation for what surgeons do now. He directed the minds of physicians and surgeons to the vital necessity of keeping wounds clean and free of contamination. Joseph Lister remains an inspiration for surgeons today. (1074 words)

collegiality /kəˈliːdʒɪˈɑːlɪtɪ/ n. 共享成果

chagrin /ˈʃæɡrɪn/ n. 懊恼

asepsis /æˈsepsɪs/ n. 无菌

sterile /ˈsteraɪl/ adj. 无菌的，消毒的

Notes:

1. compound fracture: 开放性骨折
2. a Quaker family: *Quaker* 是基督教新教的一个派别贵格会，又称教友派或者公谊会。
3. Thomas Hodgkin: 人名，英国病理学家。1832 年他报道了 7 例淋巴瘤的临床病史和尸解发现这些病例，后来该疾病以他的名字命名为霍金奇淋巴瘤。
4. house surgeon: 外科住院医生
5. Regius Professor: 多指（英国牛津、剑桥的）皇家钦定教授
6. pockets of pus: 脓袋

7. laudable pus: 黄稠脓
8. the Royal College of Surgeons: 英国皇家外科学院
9. Pasteur: 人名，法国微生物学家、化学家，他开创了微生物生理学。他发明的巴氏消毒法直至今日仍在沿用。
10. carbolic acid : 石炭酸
11. Lancet: 中文译名《柳叶刀》。该杂志是目前世界医学界最权威的学术刊物之一，也是影响因子最高的 SCI 刊物之一。
12. a Peer: (英国有权或曾经有权在上议院投票的)贵族

While You Read

Task 1: Reading Skills Practice

Directions: In critical reading, distinguishing objective facts and subjective opinions in each part or paragraph is a very important skill . (See ***Skills Bank***) . Fast read the whole text, and take notes about the main facts and the author's opinions about Joseph Lister's personal life and achievements. Then, give a 5-min oral presentation on "What I know about Joseph Lister".

	Main Ideas	Para.	Key Sentences in the Text
Facts about Joseph Lister	His Family Background		1. 2.
	His Educational Background		1. 2. 3.
	His Great Achievements		1. 2. 3. ...
Opinions about Joseph Lister	His Great Accomplishments and Imperfections		1. 2. 3. ...

Task 2: Text-related Presentation

Directions:Read carefully the part of Text B that corresponds to your task, and prepare a 1-min presentation in a unique and creative way. Remember to turn in the slip with the details of your task to your teacher before you present. (The slip can be found at the end of the book)

1) Introduce the family background of Joseph Lister and explain how it affects his career. (Para.3-Para.4)

2) Tell the class what inflammation is and its relationship with surgical infection. (Para.5)

3) Describe the world of surgery when Lister began his practice. (Para.7)

4) How old he get interest and make great breakthrough in wound cave? (Para.7-Para.9)

5) Introduce Pasteur and his germ theory and its relationship with Lister's antiseptic approach? (Para.9)

6) Introduce Listers methods of antisepsis and the modern techniques of sterilization for wound care.

After You Read

Task 1: Oral Presenting

Directions: Try to rephrase or explain the following sentences without using the boldfaced words or phrases. (This is going to be integrated into the communicative interaction in the classroom. The task can be done orally in the classroom.)

1. It was Lister's genius to **take the work** of Pasteur on the etiology of fermentation and **envision this process as the same** that was causing infection and gangrene.
2. Lister **did come to understand** that inflammation caused loss of vitality, which **rendered tissues helpless** as if they were dead, helpless against organisms he would eventually attribute as the cause of the devastating and feared surgical site infections.
3. **Operative procedures** were only occasionally performed in the average surgeon's practice, and **there was talk of banning all surgery from hospitals** because of septic complications.
4. He began **his antiseptic method** with compound fracture wounds because the standard treatment of amputation was always available **should his method fail**.
5. Although his students had the utmost respect and praise for him, **collegiality in Glasgow was a problem**, and he neglected to share credit for his success with other members of the Glasgow team, **to the great chagrin of** the Royal Infirmary administration.

Task 2: Critical Thinking

Directions: Work in groups and discuss the following question. At the end of your discussion, each group will make a list of your key points in the table and select a reporter to present your opinions. The group members should take turns to report and take notes in this semester.

From Lister's story, we have got some ideas about the history and development of surgery. Please discuss from a medical professional's view about Joseph Lister's great contributions to modern surgery.

After-class Tasks

Task 1: Word Chunks

Directions: Complete the following word chunks taken from Text A and Text B according to their Chinese equivalents and make a sentence with each word chunk.

1. ________ fractures 开放性骨折
2. ________surgery 内腔外科手术
3. loss of________精神萎靡
4. ________ of blood vessel 血栓
5. wound ________伤口愈合
6. ________ diseases 传染性疾病
7. ________ of the air 空气饱和
8. ________ method 抗菌法
9. ________ technique 无菌法
10. free of________无污染
11. ________ rate 死亡率
12. ________ rate 发病率
13. ________ stone 膀胱结石
14. intestinal ________肠梗阻
15. ________ diagnosis 定位诊断
16. ________anatomy 病理解剖学
17. heart________ 心力衰竭
18. ________ physiology 实验生理学
19. ________ medicine 内科
20. ________ hemostasis 术中止血

Task 2: Translation

Directions: Translate sentence 1 to 3 into Chinese and pay close attention to the translation of the words in bold. Then translate sentence 4 to 6 into English using the words in the bracket.

1. With the breathtaking advances made in **pathologic anatomy** and **experimental physiology** during the 18th and first part of the 19th centuries, physicians would soon adopt **a therapeutic viewpoint** that had long been prevalent among surgeons.

____

____

2. **On the centenary of** Joseph Lister's death, it is appropriate to remember and honor his **remarkable accomplishments** that earned him the title"father of modern surgery."

____

____

3. His **main research interest** was inflammation, a process then considered a specific disease and not **a response by healthy tissues to infection**.

____

____

4. 在过去，外科医生只能处理简单的骨折、脱臼和脓肿，偶尔能熟练地进行截肢手术，但是病人的死亡率却很高。(with dexterity)

____

____

5. 利斯特开始抗菌探索时，按照今天的标准，当时的外科水平还非常落后。(be primitive)

____

____

6. 利斯特也是人，历史适当地记载了他的一些不完美之处。(duly)

____

____

Task 3: Listening & Speaking

Directions: Watch the video and finish the guided note-taking before making an oral summary of what have learnt from the video.

Word Bank

transplant /træns'plɑːnt/ v. 移植　　delegate /'delɪgət/ n. 代表，团队

1) Tasks that surgeons have:

____

2) Challenges faced by the surgeons:

Before operations:

____

During operations:

____

After operations:

---

3) Basic requirements of being a surgeon:

Task 4: Research

Directions: Do some research into "*surgical achievements of the last 50 years*" and decide within your group which one is the most significant for the development of surgery. Then brainstorm the following aspects in groups before you develop your discussions into an oral presentation for the next class. You can present in the form of an interview, short play or simply a lecture. Make sure each member of the group will present his or her part on the stage.

1) What were the initial techniques used in this area?

2) What was the turning point in this area of surgery?

3) How did the solution change human life?

4) Who made the contributions to this achievement and how did he come up with the idea?

Resources

Here are the websites where you can find the useful information for your research.

http://www.nejm.org/doi/full/10.1056/NEJMra1202392

http://www.slucare.edu/pdf_nov5/history_surgery.pdf

http://www.bbc.co.uk/schools/gcsebitesize/history/shp/modern/indrevsurgeryrev1.shtml

Task 5: Writing

Directions: Write a summary of **Joseph Lister: Father of Modern Surgery.** Make sure you fully understand the text and have basic skills of writing summary before summarizing it.

Task 6: Vocabulary Log

Directions: Please finish the vocabulary log (Please find the log at the end of the book) by looking up the dictionary and write down the words or expressions you have learned in this unit by following the examples already listed in the log. And then write down the translation for each vocabulary item and if possible, its variants, synonym, antonym and the frequent collocations.

Task 7: Reading Log

Directions: After learning the whole unit and conducting the research, you have known more about surgery from different perspectives. You can go to the library or surf on the internet for more knowledge about it. You can take down the key information according to the sample chart.(Please find the chart at the end of the book) Also you are allowed to complete the chart on a computer or tablet so that this section is expandable if you want to write more than the space on a paper form might allow. And then send it to your teacher by emails. The reading log can serve as an informal way to keep track of your reading progress.

Unit 6

Future of Surgery

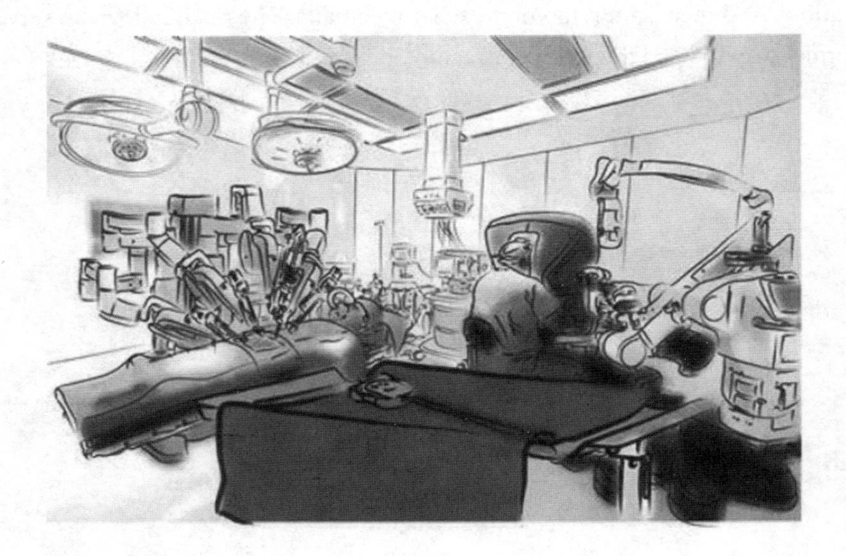

Surgeons must be very careful
When they take the knife!
Underneath their fine incisions
Stirs the culprit—Life!

——Emily Elizabeth Dickinson

Skills Bank

Deducing Meaning of Unfamiliar Lexical Items

As part of the process of learning to read, students will encounter unfamiliar or unknown words. Students can use context clues such as visuals, synonyms, antonyms, definitions and examples to help guess the meaning of unfamiliar or unknown words.

There are three tips to help readers to guess the meaning of difficult words:

1. Consider visuals such as photographs, illustrations, graphs or charts. Readers can use the visual cues found in drawings or photographs in their books and reading selections to help them guess meaning. They can do the same with more complex graphics.

2. Look for synonyms or antonyms in the sentence. Search the sentence for words that might mean the same as, or the opposite of, the unknown word. Writers sometimes use synonyms or antonyms as context clues.

3. Search for explanations or examples in the sentence or in the sentences around it. Look for a phrase that might define the unknown word. The writer might also include examples to help the reader with the meaning of the unfamiliar word.

Pre-class Tasks

Task 1: Medical Terminology Study

Directions: Study the word roots, prefixes and suffixes listed in the table below and do the **Vocabulary Preview** exercise for Text A or/ and Text B according to your teacher's instructions.

Roots	Meaning
tom/o	section 部分，断层
path/o	disease 疾病
palp/o, palpat/o	to touch gently 轻轻触碰
lapar/o	abdominal wall; abdomen 腹壁，腹部
gynec/o	woman; female 妇科
ot/o	ear 耳

续表

Roots	Meaning
laryng/o	larynx (voice box) 声带
adrenal/o	adrenal gland 肾上腺
prostat/o	prostate gland 前列腺
hyster/o	uterus; womb 子宫
sangu/i	blood 血
myel/o	spinal cord; bone marrow 脊髓
mening/o	membranes covering the spinal cord & brain 脊膜
Prefixes	**Meaning**
ana-	apart 分裂
ex-	out 出去
Suffixes	**Meaning**
-graphy	process of recording 描记法；照相术
-scope	devices for looking at or discovering and measuring things 镜
-logy	study of 学科
-ectomy	removal; excision; resection 切除
-osis	condition, usually abnormal 疾病
-cele	hernia 疝气；脱肠
-tomy	process of cutting 切

Task 2: Prepared Individual Presentation

Directions: The assigned students need to prepare a 1-min oral presentation concerning the questions in **Text-related Presentation** for Text A and/or Text B as required by your teacher.

Task 3: The Muddiest Points

Directions: Read Text A and Text B in the study group to find out the sentences that are the least clear to you after your discussions, the viewpoints that you disagree with and the understanding you have achieved through discussions and the questions you want to put forward concerning the content of the texts. Put the above information in a slip and send it to the teacher via WeChat 24 hours prior to the class. (The slip can be found on the last page of the book.)

Text A

Before You Read

Task 1: Vocabulary Preview

Directions: Divide the following words into their word parts and then give their Chinese translations by referring to **Medical Terminology Study**.

Medical Terms	Prefix	Word Root(s)	Suffix	Chinese
tomography				
pathology				
palpate				
laparoscope				
gynecology				
otolaryngology				
anastomosis				
myelomeningocele				
hysterotomy				
exsanguination				
prostatectomy				
adrenalectomy				

Task 2: Warming-up

Directions: Watch the video carefully and try to answer the questions below. While watching the video, please take notes in the blanks to help you follow the content.

1) How many technologies are mentioned in the video? What are they?

2) Can you give some key words to describe these technologies in the video?

Notes

Text A Emerging Technology in Surgery

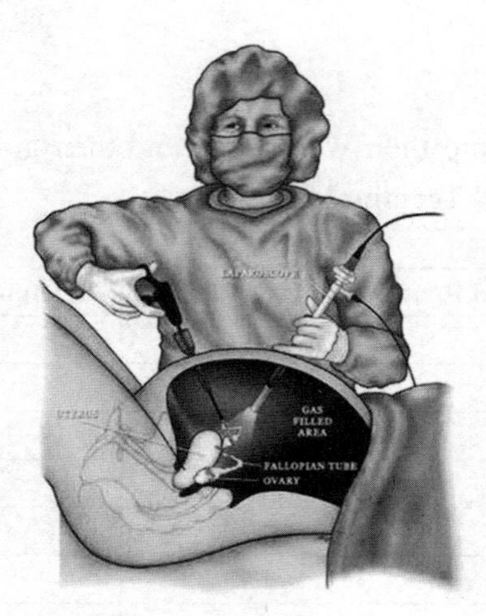

Laparoscopic surgery

1. **Laparoscopic** surgery involves the placement of a small telescope into the body cavity. The telescope **illuminates** the target tissues and conveys a bright **magnified**, high-definition image to the surgeon through an attached or incorporated camera system. The view is startling in its clarity. It eliminates shadows and affords all members of the operating team the identical view of the surgery. An important limitation of laparoscopic imaging is that it is generally **monocular** compared with the **binocular** view in open surgery, because traditional telescopes have a single-lens system. With a monocular optical system, the surgeon obtains a two-dimensional view of the body displayed on a video monitor. Other cues must be developed to appreciate the relative positions of the instruments and visualized tissues in three dimensions.

laparoscope /ˈlæpərəˌskəʊp/ n. 腹腔镜

illuminate /ɪˈluːmɪneɪt/ v. 照亮

magnified /ˈmægnɪfaɪd/ adj. 放大的

monocular /mɒˈnɒkjʊlə/ adj. 单眼的

binocular /baiˈnɔkjulə/ adj. 双眼的

2. Laparoscopic images give the surgeon a view of the surface of tissues. In open surgery, the surgeon can palpate and compress tissues to gain a sense of the presence of the **pathology** that lies deep to the surface. Because direct **manual** evaluation is not available during laparoscopy, the surgeon must adopt other methods to evaluate the tissues beneath the surface. Some of this information can be acquired before surgery by assessing the patient with cross-sectional imaging, such as ultrasound, computed **tomography** (CT), and magnetic resonance imaging (MRI). Digital CT and MR images can be displayed in the operating room using surface markers to help the surgeon consolidate these findings with the visual display of the tissue surface during surgery. An advantage of ultrasound is that it is easy to use **intraoperatively** and can be positioned to provide real-time information of the tissue being viewed through the laparoscope. A surgeon proficient in intraoperative ultrasound can incorporate the surface and cross-sectional information to evaluate the target tissues carefully.

pathology /pəˈθɒlədʒɪ/ n. 病理
manual /ˈmænjuəl/ adj. 手工的
tomography /təˈmɒgrəfɪ/ n. X线断层照相术
intraoperative /ɪntrəˈɒpərətɪv/ adj. 手术（期）中的

3. A drawback of laparoscopy is the limited field of view; the laparoscope must be moved to maintain an ideal image. The closer the laparoscope image is to the target, the better the illumination, magnification, and image detail, but the field of view is more limited. Constant communication between the surgeon performing the operation and the assistant managing the telescope is essential for safe surgery.

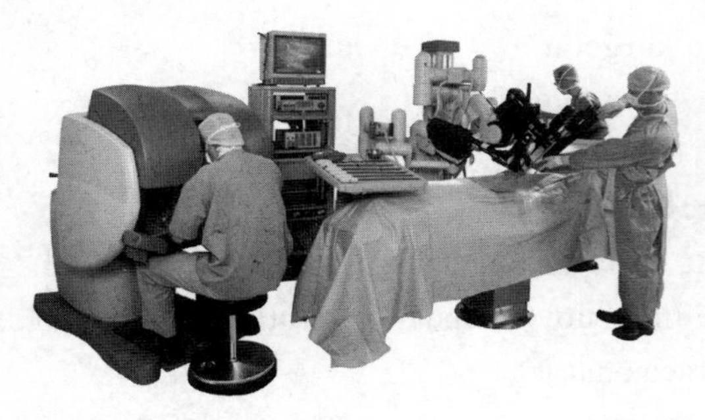

Robotic Surgery

4. The concept of robotic surgery is to use the enabling characteristics of robots to improve the capabilities of the surgeon compared with working freehand. Unlike the use of robotics in industry, the robot does not work autonomously in most surgical applications, but acts as an interface between the operating surgeon and patient. In this master-slave relationship, the master (surgeon) sits at a console, in an **ergonomic** and comfortable position, and uses movements of both hands and feet to control movement of the laparoscope and instruments (slave) in the patient. The commercially available robotic system uses a **proprietary** laparoscope with two optical systems providing binocular (three-dimensional) vision. The surgical instruments are wristed near their distal tips, so the movements of the surgeon's hands can be reproduced by the instruments without the usual limitations of the fulcrum effect[1] seen with traditional laparoscopic instruments. The degrees of freedom of the instrument are increased, making it easier to carry out fine **maneuvers** than with

ergonomic /ˌɜːgəˈnɒmɪk/ adj. 人类工程学的

proprietary /prəˈpraɪətri/ adj. 所有人的

maneuver /məˈnuːvə/ n. 移动

traditional laparoscopic surgery. The surgeon can work from within the operating room or even remotely because there is no direct contact between the surgeon at the **console** and the instruments. One consequence of this interface is that the surgeon has no **tactile** sense of the tissues, but must adapt by using visual information.

console /kən'səʊl/ n.（机器的）控制台

tactile /'tæktaɪl/ adj. 有触感的

5. Robotic surgery has opened up the concept of telesurgery. Theoretically, the surgeon can operate on patients at great distance. Before this can be applied practically, issues of licensing and liability must be addressed, and **latent** delays between motion of the surgeon and movement of the instrument must be resolved. The longer the distance that the data needs to be transmitted from the console to the patient, the greater the latent delay. Delays of more than 250 milliseconds can have a significant impact on the quality of the surgery. Robotic surgical platforms are appealing for support of the injured soldier and of patients in hostile environments, such as outer space missions, deep sea exploration, and polar expeditions.

latent /'leɪtnt/ adj. 潜在的

6. Currently, minimally invasive surgery robotic systems are widely used in **urologic** surgery and **gynecology** and, to a lesser extent in cardiac surgery, **otolaryngology**, and general surgery. The main drawbacks are the costs, bulkiness, setup time for the equipment, and absence of **compelling** data to show superiority of robotic operations over those

urologic /jʊərəʊ'lɒdʒɪk/ adj. 泌尿道的

gynecology /ˌgaɪnɪ'kɒlədʒɪ/ n. 妇产科学

otolaryngology /ˌəʊtəʊlærɪŋ'gɒlədʒi/ n. 耳鼻喉科学

compelling /kəm'pelɪŋ/ adj. 不可抗拒的，有说服力的

done by well-trained laparoscopic surgeons. Recently, robotic surgery has been carried out in conjunction with robotic-assisted anesthesia. This is an automated platform on which anesthesia agents are controlled using computer-assisted devices that calculate moment-to-moment anesthesia doses in a closed-loop system[2] to provide optimal dosing. (791 words)

Notes:

1. fulcrum effect: 支点效应
2. closed-loop system: 闭环系统，是由信号正向通路和反馈通路构成闭合回路的自动控制系统，又称反馈控制系统。

While You Read

Task: Text-related Presentation

Directions:Read carefully the part of Text A that corresponds to your task, and prepare a 1-min presentation in a unique and creative way. Remember to turn in the slip with the details of your task to your teacher before you present. (The slip can be found at the end of the book)

1. Explain how laparoscopic surgery works. (Para. 2)
2. Talk about the advantages and disadvantages of laparoscopic surgery. (Para.2-Para.4)
3. Explain how robotic surgery works together with surgeons. (Para. 5)
4. Talk about the advantages and disadvantages of robotic surgery. (Para. 6)

After You Read

Task 1: Academic English Study

Directions: Read this section carefully and try to find more examples of nominalization in Text A and Text B.

Complexity (IV)

Nominalization

Another way to make academic English more complex than general English is the use of nominalization.

Formal written English uses nouns more than verbs. For example, "judgement" rather than "judge", "development" rather than "develop", "admiration" rather than "admire". Changing a verb or other word into a noun is called nominalization.

Instead of:

This information enables us to formulate precise questions.

we would write:

This information enables the formulation of precise questions.

More examples are:

Ex: Because direct manual *evaluation* is not available during laparoscopy, the surgeon must adopt other methods to evaluate the tissues beneath the surface. (Para.2)

Ex: The closer the laparoscope image is to the target, the better the *illumination, magnification*, and image detail, but the field of view is more limited. (Para.3)

Task 2: Critical Thinking

Directions: Work in groups and discuss the following question. At the end of your discussion, each group will assign a representative to present your opinions on this issue.

Surgical mistakes happen more commonly than people think. One in every three thousand surgeries will result in something being left in the body of the patient. The robotic surgeons also are found making mistakes either because of the malfunction of the machines or the unprofessional conduct of surgeons in control of the robotic machines. But not all mistakes can cost the life of a patient. If a patient makes a full recovery, should doctors admit to a mistake that might have otherwise gone unnoticed? What if the patient looks at an admission of error as a winning ticket in the malpractice lottery?

Text B

Before You Read

Task 1: Vocabulary Preview

Directions: Preview the words in the table below and use them to describe the following pictures.

laparoscopy anastomosis console manipulator hysterotomy adrenalectomy

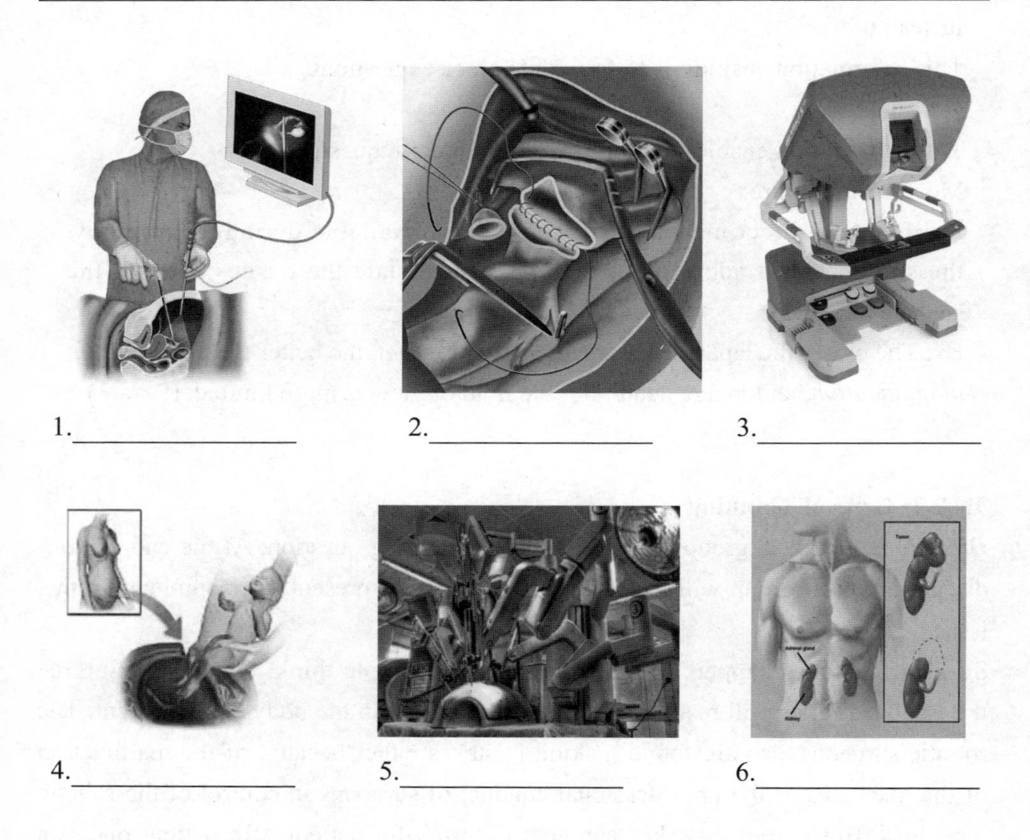

1.________ 2.________ 3.________

4.________ 5.________ 6.________

Task 2: Warming-up

Directions: Watch the video clip carefully and try to answer the questions below. While watching the video, please take notes in the blanks to help you follow the content.

1) What's the name of the surgical technology mentioned in the video?

2) How does it work?

3) According to the video, what are the advantages and disadvantages of this technology?

Notes

Text B Robotic Surgery — Squeezing into Tight Places

Norman T. Berlinger, M.D., Ph.D.

1. Back in the 1980s, the **rationale** for building a surgical robot was the stuff of science fiction. Intent on providing "a doctor in every **foxhole**," military strategists envisioned a severely wounded soldier being loaded into a battlefield ambulance equipped with a robot so that a surgeon at a Mobile Army Surgical Hospital[1], or MASH unit, miles away could perform life-saving telesurgery to prevent **exsanguination** or some other physiological **catastrophe**. The National Aeronautics and Space Administration[2] had a similar vision. A **terrestrial** physician would be able to remove an acutely inflamed appendix from a patient aboard a robot-equipped space

rationale /ˌræʃəˈnɑːl/ n. 基本理论

foxhole /ˈfɒkshəʊl/ n. 散兵坑

exsanguination /eksˈsæŋgwəneɪʃn/ n. 放血，驱血法

catastrophe /kəˈtæstrəfɪ/ n. 灾祸

terrestrial /təˈrestrɪəl/ adj. 地球的

station. In this high-tech future, surgery could be performed skillfully and promptly even in dangerous or **inaccessible** places.

inaccessible /ɪnæk'sesəbl/ adj. 达不到的

2. By the 1990s, the rationale for such robots had become even more compelling. Minimally invasive laparoscopic surgery wasn't overcoming its severest limitations. Many kinds of **anastomoses**, especially of the microscopic variety, could not be performed well, if at all[3]. Laparoscopic instruments were rigid tools that could move and rotate along only two axes (moving inward, outward, clockwise, and counterclockwise, with four "degrees of freedom") and so could not duplicate surgeons' ability to apply pitch and yaw[4] to their wrists — that is, to **tilt** manual instruments up and down or shift them from side to side. And whereas surgeons have binocular vision and rely heavily on their depth **perception**, the laparoscopic camera transmitted only a two-dimensional image. Alas, minimally invasive surgery proved to be good for **extirpation** but not for reconstruction.

anastomosis /ənæstə'məʊsɪs/ n. 吻合，连接

tilt /tɪlt/ v. 倾斜

perception /pə'sepʃn/ n. 感知

extirpation /ˌekstə'peɪʃn/ n. 摘除

3. Then, market forces **dictated** further innovations. Consumer-minded patients were demanding even more kinds of minimally invasive surgery. Insurers liked the shortened recovery periods associated with such operations, and medical-center accountants **relished** the increased flow of revenue. Hospitals began putting pictures of robots on the front of their advertising brochures.

dictate /dɪk'teɪt/ v. 支配

relish /'relɪʃ/ v. 品味，欣赏

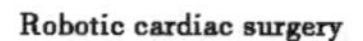

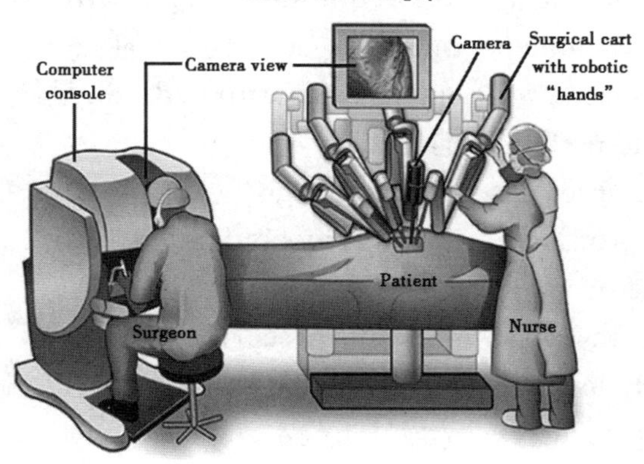

4. So what, exactly, do the current **incarnations** of surgical robots consist of? Although many have fanciful **anthropomorphic** names such as da Vinci, ZEUS, AESOP, and Robodoc, they don't look at all like humans. Unlike industrial robots, they are not autonomous, and to be **taxonomically** correct, they ought not to be called machines. A surgical robot is actually a collection of wristed "servant" tools called **manipulators**, which receive digital instructions from an interfaced computer. The "master" surgeon, seated at an ergonomically designed video console with an "**immersive**" three-dimensional display, initiates the digital instructions by controlling sophisticated hand grips — essentially, **joysticks** with seven degrees of freedom (adding the pitch, the yaw, and the "pincer-like" movement to those that were already available). The manipulators inside the patient's body duplicate the surgeon's hand movements at the console, and software filters out even physiologic hand **tremors**. More than 10,000 operations have already been performed in this way.

incarnation /ˌɪnkɑːˈneɪʃn/ n. 化身

anthropomorphic /ˌænθrəpəˈmɔːfɪk/ adj. 赋予人性的

taxonomically /ˌtæksəuˈnɔmikəlɪ/ adv. 分类学的

manipulator /məˈnɪpjuleɪtə(r)/ n. 操纵器；控制器

immersive /ɪˈmɜːsɪv/ adj. 拟真的；沉浸式的

joystick /ˈdʒɔɪstɪk/ n. 操纵杆

tremor /ˈtremə(r)/ n. 震颤；战栗

5. **Unaccommodating** places are what robot-assisted surgery is all about. The human surgeon is not **optimized** for tiny spaces. An **otolaryngologist** by trade, I used to perform microscopic middle-ear surgery in a space the size of a **pistachio** shell. Too many of these operations were struggles. Because pediatric surgeons must frequently work in small spaces, they have applied minimally invasive techniques to a broader range of procedures — such as **fundoplication** and ligation of patent ductus arteriosus[5] — than have other surgical specialists.

unaccommodating /'ʌnə'kɒmədeɪtɪŋ/ adj. 不随和的
optimized /'ɒptɪmaɪzd/ adj. 最佳的
otolaryngologist /əʊtələ'rɪŋgɒlədʒɪst/ n. 耳鼻喉科医师
pistachio /pɪ'stæʃiəʊ/ n. 开心果
fundoplication /fʌn'dɒplɪkeɪʃn/ n. 胃底折叠术

6. With the advent of robotics, pediatric surgeons began to dream about fixing fetal **diaphragmatic hernias** or **myelomeningoceles** in utero: a robot's computer can scale down a surgeon's hand movements into micromotions inside the fetal patient. And because no **hysterotomy** is required, such surgery is not subject to the disastrous complication of preterm labor.

diaphragmatic/daɪəfræg'mætɪk/ adj. 横膈膜的
hernia /hə:niə/ n. 疝，脱肠
myelomeningocele /maɪələʊmɪ'nɪŋgɒsi:l/ n. 脊髓脊膜突出
hysterotomy /'hɪstə'rɒtəmɪ/ n. 子宫切开术

7. In addition to small or narrow places in the human body, remote places in the world are often mentioned by those invoking the promise of robotic surgery. Some observers have called "Operation Lindbergh," the first transatlantic **cholecystectomy**, nothing more than theater: a telesurgeon in New York robotically removed a gallbladder from a patient in Strasbourg, France — without complications. But Krummel articulates the logical extension of this mode of operation: "Telesurgery might be a good way to distribute

cholecystectomy /ˌkɒlɪsɪs'tektəmɪ/ n. 胆囊切除术

health care in the Third World." And NASA hasn't forgotten about its potential for the proposed manned missions to the Moon and to Mars.

8. Of course, important disadvantages of the robotic approach abound. A robot can cost $1 million or more, not including the maintenance contract and the expensive disposable items required for each procedure. Each robot's footprint is quite big, and its instruments don't provide a sense of touch. Not unexpectedly, the learning curve for the effective use of these tools is long and steep. The robot's toolbox isn't very full, and the time required to switch from one instrument to another lengthens operating time. Most of all, the majority of published studies of robot-assisted surgery have really been technical notes describing **feasibility**. **Prospective** studies comparing robotic with conventional procedures will be needed in order to establish a clear benefit.

feasibility /ˌfiːzəˈbɪlətɪ/ n. 可行性
prospective /prəˈspektɪv/ adj. 前瞻性的

9. But even as the current robotic systems begin to be put to such tests, the true **visionaries** in this domain are focusing on the surgical robot less as a mechanical device than as an information system — one that should be fused with other information systems. One proposed example of this kind of fusion is image-guided surgery, also called surgical navigation. Robot-assisted surgeons will be able to see real-time, three-dimensional scanner images electronically **superimposed** over the operative field that is displayed on

visionary /ˈvɪʒənrɪ/ n. 有远见的人
superimpose /ˌsuːpərɪmˈpəʊz/ v. 重叠；添加

the monitor. In other words, on the screen, human anatomy will be rendered **translucent**, and the surgeon will be able to determine the exact location of a tumor and more readily avoid damaging vital structures. In fact, with preoperative scanner images, surgeons could robotically practice their patients' surgery the night before, and the robot's computer could be programmed not to allow its instruments to penetrate the vena cava, thereby eliminating bloody intraoperative mishaps.

translucent /træns'lu:snt/ adj. 半透明的；有光泽的

10. Surgery is going digital. It's no longer about blood and guts but bits and bytes. Surgical robotics is not an end technology, but a step along the way to something bigger. What might be a bit troubling though is that the first part of the progress curve seems long and flat. But, that's how it's been with so many other big advances. (1040 words)

Notes:

1. Mobile Army Surgical Hospital:（美国）陆军流动外科医院，简称 MASH。
2. National Aeronautics and Space Administration:（美国）国家航空航天局，简称 NASA 。
3. if at all: 就算真的有，也……（置于句末，具体意思根据句子前半部分而定）
4. pitch and yaw: 俯仰和偏航
5. ductus arteriosus: 动脉导管

While You Read

Task 1: Reading Skills Practice

Directions: Context clues such as visuals, synonyms, antonyms, examples can be used to decode the meaning of difficult new words. The clues of three new words are given in the table, please write down their Chinese according to the clues. And then find more new words and write down the clues you use to guess their meanings by referring to the ***Skills Bank***.

New Words	Chinese	Synonym/ Antonym	Explanation/ Example	Visual
relish		Insurers liked the shortened recovery periods associated with such operations, and medical-center accountants relished the increased flow of revenue.		
anthropo-morphic			Although many have fanciful anthropomorphic names such as da Vinci, ZEUS, AESOP, and Robodoc, they don't look at all like humans.	
console				1 Surgeon Console 2 Image Processing Equipment 3 Endowrist Instruments 4 Surgical Arm Cart 5 Hi-Resolution 3-D Endoscope

Task 2: Text-related Presentation

Directions:Read carefully the part of Text B that corresponds to your task, and prepare a 1-min presentation in a unique and creative way. Remember to turn in the slip with the details of your task to your teacher before you present. (The slip can be found at the end of the book)

1. Introduce the rationale for robotic surgery in 1980s. (Para. 1)
2. Introduce the rationale for robotic surgery in 1990s. (Para. 2)
3. Talk about the factors that finally put robots into the market. (Para. 3)
4. Explain how the robotic surgery works together with the telesurgeon. (Para. 4)
5. Illustrate with examples the advantages and disadvantages of robotic surgery. (Para. 5-Para. 10)

After You Read

Task 1: Oral Presenting

Directions: Try to rephrase or explain the following sentences without using the boldfaced words or phrases.(This is going to be integrated into the communicative interaction in the classroom. The task can be done orally in the classroom.)

1. **Unlike** the use of robotics in industry, the robot does not work **autonomously** in most surgical applications, but **acts as an interface** between the operating surgeon and patient.
2. The rate of growth and the potential for **merging** many of these technologies **holds great promise for** patient safety and for **delivering** surgical care, with its values of effective and durable treatment, at a much lower cost to the patient **in terms of** pain and suffering.
3. **Intent on** providing "a doctor in every foxhole," military strategists **envisioned** a severely wounded soldier being loaded into a battlefield ambulance equipped with a robot so that a surgeon at a Mobile Army Surgical Hospital, or MASH unit, miles away could perform life-saving telesurgery to prevent exsanguination or some other physiological catastrophe.
4. The "master" surgeon, seated at an ergonomically designed video console with an "immersive" three-dimensional display, **initiates the digital instructions** by controlling **sophisticated** hand grips — essentially, joysticks with seven degrees of freedom (adding the pitch, the yaw, and the "pincer-like" movement to those that were already available).

5. The robot-assisted procedure is **associated with** lower rates of postoperative impotence and incontinence than the open procedure because the robot makes it considerably easier to **spare** nerves and to anastomose the urethra.

Task 2: Critical Thinking

Directions: Work in groups and discuss the following questions. At the end of your discussion, each group will assign a representative to present your points on this issue.

Robots are popping up in operating rooms around the world. The da Vinci Surgical System robot is now used in four out of five prostatectomies in the United States, and more than 1800 of the machines are installed at some 1400 hospitals worldwide. Although today's robots are still controlled by surgeons, some researchers say that may not be the case in the future. Bioengineers at Duke University, in Durham, N.C., have demonstrated that an autonomous robot can perform simple surgery, such as taking a sample of a cyst, on its own. Since then, other researchers have wondered whether fully autonomous robots could perform more complicated tasks.

Do you think robots will one day replace surgeons for certain procedures? Would you trust a robot over a surgeon?

After-class Tasks

Task 1: Collocations

Directions: Complete the following word chunks taken from Text A and Text B according to their Chinese equivalents and make a sentence with each word chunk.

1. ________ target issue 照亮目标组织
2. convey ________ image 传递高清图像
3. ________ shadow 消除阴影
4. ________ information 横断面信息
5. ________ ultrasound 术中超声
6. ________ surgeons 训练有素的医生
7. a ________ soldier 严重受伤的士兵
8. a ________ appendix 严重发炎的阑尾
9. ________ surgery 微创手术
10. ________ surgery 机器人辅助手术
11. ________ surgeon 小儿外科医生
12. the ________ of robotics 机器人技术的到来
13. determine the ________ of a tumor 确定肿瘤位置
14. penetrate the ________ 渗入腔静脉
15. eliminate ________ 消除术中意外
16. shorten the ________ 缩短康复时间
17. ________ imaging 横断面图像
18. ________ technology 终结技术
19. complication of ________ 早产并发症
20. ________ the gallbladder 移除胆囊

Task 2: Translation

Directions: Translate sentence 1 to 3 into Chinese and pay close attention to the translation of words in bold. Then translate sentence 4 to 6 into English using the words in the bracket.

1. Military strategists **envisioned** a severely wounded soldier being loaded into a battlefield ambulance equipped with a robot so that a surgeon at a Mobile Army Surgical Hospital could perform life-saving telesurgery to prevent exsanguination or some other **physiological catastrophe**.

____

____

2. The telescope **illuminates** the target tissues and conveys a bright **magnified**, **high-definition image** to the surgeon through an **attached or incorporated** camera system.

____

____

3. The main drawbacks are the costs, bulkiness, setup time for the equipment, and **absence of compelling data** to show **superiority** of robotic operations over those done by well-trained laparoscopic surgeons.

____

____

4. 引入抗菌消毒法和麻醉使得外科手术实现了现代化。(with the introduction of)

____

____

5. 与全麻相比，局部麻醉可以降低术后发病率、死亡率、住院时间及成本。(compared with)

____

____

6. 白内障通常病情进展缓慢，就算要手术也要过很多年。(if at all)

____

____

Task 3: Listening & Speaking

Directions: Watch the video carefully and take down notes under the three subtitles listed below. Then present the three parts with the help of the notes.

Word Bank

prickly /'prɪklɪ/ ad. 棘手的
hollow /'hɑləʊ/ ad. 空的
tubular /'tjubjʊlə/ ad. 管状的
miniature / 'mɪnətʃə/ n. 缩图

1. Implications of 3D printing in modern medicine

____

____

2. Difficulties of organ printing

____

____

3. Body on a chip project and its goals

____

____

Task 4: Research

Directions: Do some research on *how the robotic technology affects the future young surgeons. You can include their medical education, their roles in the surgery and their relationship with the patients and machines.* You can present in the form of an interview, short play or simply a lecture. Make sure each member of the group will present his or her part on the stage.

Resources

http://www.sld.cu/galerias/pdf/uvs/cirured/estres_y_cirugia.pdf
http://www.ncbi.nlm.nih.gov/pubmed/15476646

Task 5: Writing

Directions: Write an essay titled ***Robot-assisted Surgery versus Conventional Open Surgery***. You can compare or contrast the two approaches from the following aspects by referring to the content in Text A and Text B and also by doing more research: the inherent technology (the merits and disadvantages), the doctor's perspective (learning curve and adaptation, etc.), the patients' perspective(acceptance of new technology) and other dimensions such as the economic factor.

Task 6: Vocabulary Log

Directions: Please finish the vocabulary log (Please find the log at the end of the book) by looking up the dictionary and write down the words or expressions you have learnt in this unit by following the examples already listed in the log. And then write down the translation for each vocabulary item and if possible, its variants, synonym, antonym and the frequent collocations.

Task 7: Reading Log

Directions: After learning the whole unit and conducting the research, you have known more about recent surgical development from different perspectives. You can go to the library or surf on the internet for more knowledge about it. You can take down the key information according to the sample chart. (Please find the chart at the end of the book) Also you are allowed to complete the chart on a computer or tablet so that this section is expandable if you want to write more than the space on a paper form might allow. And then send it to your teacher by emails. The reading log can serve as an informal way to keep track of your reading progress.

Unit 7

Awareness of Anesthesia

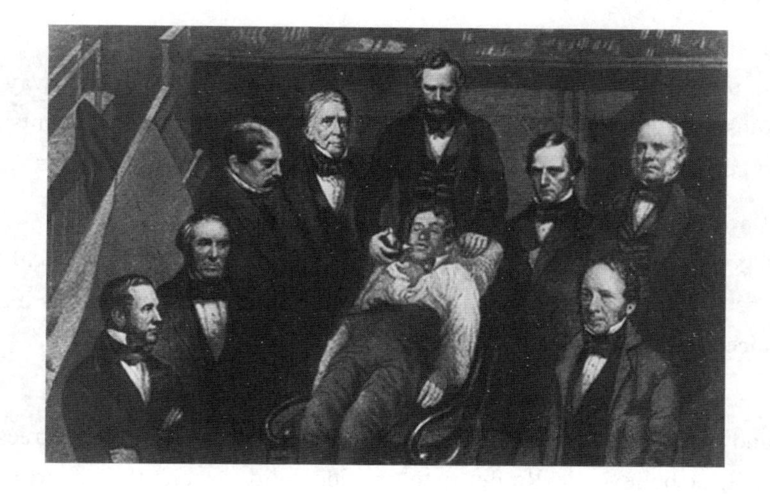

The effect was soothing, quieting & delightful beyond measure.

——Queen Victoria

Skills Bank

Recognizing Valid and Invalid Arguments

When authors use logical reasoning in their passages, they are said to contain valid arguments. These arguments are based upon facts and accurate details. Conversely, when authors use illogical reasoning in their passages, they are said to contain invalid arguments. Invalid arguments are based on some type of faulty reasoning, called fallacies.

Fallacies that rely on irrelevant issues and/or emotional appeals:

1. Ad Hominem (argument to the person)

Authors use ad hominem when they shift the focus of an argument away from the issues and towards the authors' opponent. Ad hominem arguments often contain personal commentary and personal attacks.

2. Ad Populum (argument to the people)

The ad populum fallacy occurs when authors evade the issues and appeal to the emotions of the people-the reader in this case. The authors' appeal is made to allegiances and beliefs that people hold dear.

3. Bandwagon Appeal

The bandwagon appeal appears when authors suggest that everyone agrees with it, does it, or believes it. Rather than provide solid reasons to support claims, the author merely suggests that since everyone else is in agreement it is valid support-BUT IT IS NOT!

4. Red Herring

Authors sometimes introduce irrelevant issues to distract the reader's attention away from the real issues. This is the red herring fallacy. You can easily remember the "red herring" fallacy if you remember how the term originated. During foxhunts, servants would drag a smoked herring fish across the trail of the foxes. The fish scent would divert the hunting dogs' attention away from the foxes and lengthened the "thrill of the chase" for the hunters. Likewise, when authors use red herring fallacy, they divert your attention away from the real issues.

Pre-class Tasks

Task 1: Medical Terminology Study

Directions: Study the word roots, prefixes and suffixes listed in the table below and do the **Vocabulary Preview** exercise for Text A or/ and Text B according to your teacher's instructions.

Roots	Meaning
esthesia esthesi/o	nervous sensation 神经感觉
hal	breathe 呼吸
ven/o ven/i	vein 静脉血管
vas/o	vessel; duct 血管
dur/o	dura mater 硬脑（脊）膜
trach/	trachea (windpipe) 气管
lapar/o	abdominal wall; abdomen 腹部
chol/e	bile, gall 胆
cyst/o	urinary bladder; cyst; sac of fluid 膀胱；囊
cardi/o	heart 心脏
cis/o	cut 切
Prefix	**Meaning**
a(an)-	no, not, without 没有
in-	in; into 里面
intra-	within, into 在……内
epi-	above; upon; on 在……上
para-	near; beside; abnormal; apart from; along the side of 旁边
tacky-	fast 快
Suffix	**Meaning**
-ia	condition 疾病
-tomy	process of cutting 切除
-ician	specialist 专家
-scope	instrument for visual examination 检查或观察用镜
-al/-ac	pertaining to 与……有关
-lysis	breakdown; separation; destruction; loosening 崩溃，分开，损坏

Task 2: Prepared Individual Presentation

Directions: The assigned students need to prepare a 1-min oral presentation concerning the questions in **Text-related Presentation** for Text A and/or Text B as required by your teacher.

Task 3: The Muddiest Points

Directions: Read Text A and Text B in the study group to find out the sentences that are the least clear to you after your discussions, the viewpoints that you disagree with and the understanding you have achieved through discussions and the questions you want to put forward concerning the content of the texts. Put the above information in a slip and send it to the teacher via WeChat 24 hours prior to the class. (The slip can be found on the last page of the book.)

In-class Tasks

Text A

Before You Read

Task 1: Vocabulary Preview

Directions: Divide the following words into their word parts and then give their Chinese translations based on the table above.

Medical Terms	Prefix	Word Root(s)	Suffix	Chinese
anesthesia				
inhalation				
intravenous				
vasectomy				
epidural				
incision				
anesthesiologist				
laparoscopic				
cholecystectomy				
tachycardia				
arrhythmia				
paralyze				

Task 2: Warming-up

Directions: Watch the video carefully and try to answer the questions below. While watching the video, please take notes in the blanks to help you follow the content.

1) When was the first anesthetic surgery performed in history according to the video?

2) How many kinds of anesthesia are mentioned in the video? What are they?

Notes

Text A The Practice of Anesthesia

1. Over the years there have been many inventions which have made our lives easier. Considering these inventions, perhaps none is as overlooked as **anesthesia**.

anesthesia /ˌænəsˈθiːʒə/ n. 麻醉

2. The term anesthesia is defined as the loss of sensitivity to pain brought about by various drugs (**anesthetics**). It is used during many medical procedures, including surgical procedures. The type of anesthesia to adopt depends on the procedure being performed and the physical and emotional status of the patient.

anesthetic /ˌænəsˈθetɪk/ n. 麻醉剂

General Anesthesia

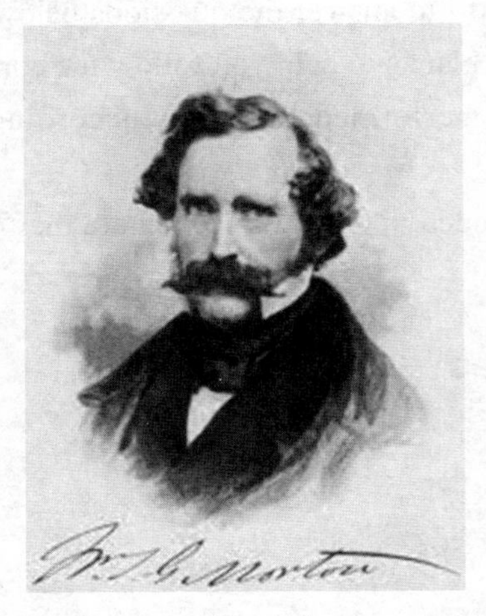

3. William T. G. Morton[1] became the first to publicly demonstrate the use of **diethyl ether** in October 1846 as a general anesthetic at Massachusetts General Hospital[2], in what is known today as the Ether Dome. General anesthesia is a drug-induced, **reversible** state of unconsciousness, loss of memory, pain relief and relaxation of muscles. Because it carries a higher risk for complications than other types of anesthesia, general anesthesia is used primarily for procedures that cannot be done utilizing other methods and for patients who prefer to be asleep during surgery.

diethyl ether /dai'eθil 'iːθə/ n. 乙醚，二乙醚

reversible /rɪ'vɜːsəbl/ adj. 可恢复原状的

4. A typical general anesthetic given for gallbladder removal goes as follows.

5. Oxygen is **administered** constantly, initially with a mask over the face. All the patient's bodily functions are carefully controlled and monitored. First an **intravenous** injection of **propofol** to make the patient unconscious is given. This is followed by a muscle **relaxant** given to relax muscles of the abdomen to

administer /əd'mɪnɪstə(r)/ v. 施用药物

intravenous /ˌɪntrə'viːnəs/ adj. 注入静脉的

propofol /prə'pɔːfɒl/ n. 异丙酚

relaxant /rɪ'læksənt/ n. 松弛药

place a breathing tube and to ease the surgery. A morphine-like painkiller is now injected. A mixture of anesthetic gases (which always includes oxygen) is given through the breathing tube to keep the patient unconscious throughout the whole surgery.

6. A mechanical breathing machine, called a **ventilator**, is attached. At the end of the operation, the effect of the muscle relaxants is reversed with two other drugs, and the anesthetic gases discontinued. When the patient is conscious and able to breathe without help, the ventilator is stopped and the breathing tube removed. All intravenous drugs and anesthetic gases are administered in appropriate amounts so that the patient is completely unconscious during the surgery, but awake and pain free at the end.

ventilator /'ventɪleɪtə(r)/ n. 呼吸机

Local Anesthesia

7. Local anesthesia refers to temporarily **numbing** a small area by injecting local anesthetic into the skin so that minor procedures can be done painlessly. For example, if a surgical procedure is performed on the right hand, a local anesthetic is used to numb that hand without affecting any other part of the body. This type of anesthesia is generally used for minor surgeries (e.g. breast **biopsies**, **vasectomies**) and to stitch small wounds. It is usually administered by injection, which can be painful. However, the discomfort only lasts for a brief moment and the anesthesia usually takes effect very quickly. Sometimes local anesthesia is

numb /nʌm/ v. 使失去知觉

biopsy /'baɪɒpsɪ/ n. 活组织检查（从身体取下细胞或组织进行检验）

vasectomy /və'sektəmɪ/ n. 输精管切除术

applied **topically**, as a spray or a cream. Cocaine is used medically as a sprayed anesthetic to numb the inside of the nose and throat. For the removal of a growth on the surface of the skin, an anesthetic cream can be applied to numb the area. In minimally invasive procedures that can be completed in a few minutes, an injection of local anesthesia is all that is used. More involved operations require **sedation** with the anesthesia to make the patient more comfortable and the injection more tolerable. Sedatives relax the patient and induce **drowsiness**, but they do not put patients into a deep sleep. They are usually administered by injection or through an intravenous (IV), but can be given orally or by **rectal suppository**, particularly in children.

topically /'tɒpɪkəlɪ/ adv. 局部地

sedation /sɪ'deɪʃn/ n. 药物镇静

drowsiness /'draʊzɪnəs/ n. 嗜睡

rectal suppository /'rekt(ə)l sə'pɔzitəri/ n. 直肠栓剂

Regional Anesthesia

8. Regional anesthesia involves injecting local anesthetics close to a nerve or nerves that supplies feeling (and function) to the area of the body involved in the operation. The skin and tissues that the needle goes through are also numbed with local anesthetic so that there is minimal discomfort associated with placement of the needle. Local anesthetic drugs stop nerves from working temporarily, so that no sensation and movement in the area of the body supplied by the nerve(s) occurs. This type of anesthesia is also called a nerve block. Regional anesthesia numbs a large area, or region, of the body and is used for more extensive and

invasive surgery. Regional anesthesia is often used for procedures involving the lower part of the body, such as cesarean section[2], **prostate** surgery, and operations on the legs. For example, if regional anesthesia is used for prostate surgery, the patient is numb from his navel to his toes. Some patients feel pressure or tugging during surgery performed under regional anesthesia. (756 words)

prostate /'prɒsteɪt/ n. 前列腺

Notes:

1. William Thomas Green Morton: 人名，美国麻醉医生，吸入式麻醉的发明者。
2. Cesarean section: 剖腹产

While You Read

Task: Text-related Presentation

Directions: *Read carefully the part of Text A that corresponds to your task, and prepare* a 1-min presentation in a unique and creative way. Remember to turn in the slip with the details of your task to your teacher before you present. (The slip can be found at the end of the book)

1) Before modern anesthesia was introduced into surgical procedures, how did ancient people deal with the pain in the surgery?

2) Tell us about Morton and his first public demonstration of surgery with ether. (Para.3)

3) Make comparison and contrast among local, regional and general anesthesia. (Para.4-Para.8)

After You Read

Task 1: Academic English Study

Directions: Read this section carefully and try to find more examples of objectivity in Text A and Text B.

Objectivity

This means that the main emphasis should be on the information that you want to give and the arguments you want to make, rather than you. Nobody really wants to know what you "think" or "believe". They want to know what you have studied and learned and how this has led you to your various conclusions. The thoughts and beliefs should be based on your lectures, reading, discussion and research and it is important to make this clear.

1. In general, avoid words like "I", "me", and "myself".

A reader will normally assume that any idea not referenced is your own. It is therefore unnecessary to make this explicit.

Don't write:" In my opinion, this a very interesting study."

Write: "This is a very interesting study."

Avoid "you" to refer to the reader or people in general.

2. Use more passive voice to highlight the receiver of the action and to keep the words objective

Often in academic English, we don't want to focus on who is doing an action, but on who is receiving or experiencing the action. The passive voice allows writers to highlight the most important participants or events within sentences by placing them at the beginning of the sentence. Passive voice can also avoid the use of informal personal pronouns to keep the text objective.

Ex: General anesthesia *is used* primarily for procedures that *cannot be done* utilizing other methods and for patients who prefer to be asleep during surgery.

Ex: Spinal anesthesia *is injected* into the spinal fluid with a special needle that penetrates the spinal column through the back.

Task 2: Critical Thinking

Directions: Work in groups and discuss the following question. At the end of your discussion, each group will assign a representative to present your opinions on this issue.

Suppose you decide to take a gastroscopy examination to see if there's anything wrong with your stomach. It's not an uncommon practice to take the examination without being anesthetized. In this case, you have to bear the discomfort and possible pain of the procedure. Another option is intravenous anesthesia, which can relieve pain but may be accompanied by side effects and complications. So what would you do in this situation?

Text B

Before You Read

Task 1: Vocabulary Preview

Directions: Preview the words in the table below and use them to describe the following pictures.

monitor intravenous lines laparoscopic cholecystectomy tachycardia paddle anesthetic pump

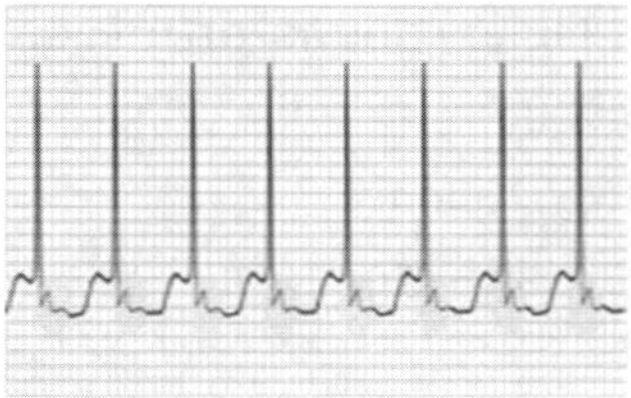

1.________________ 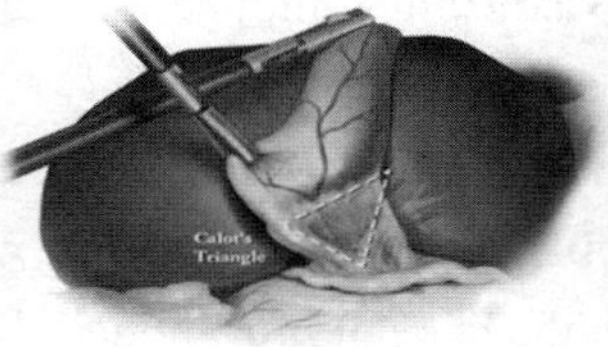 2.________________ 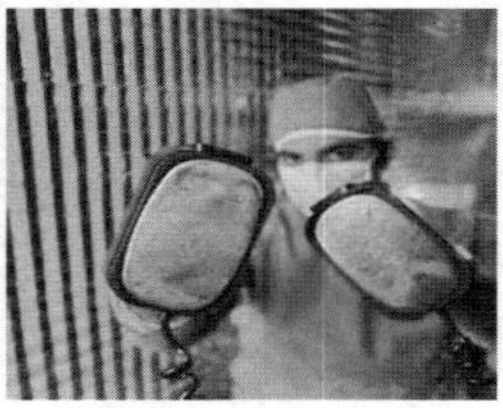 3.________________

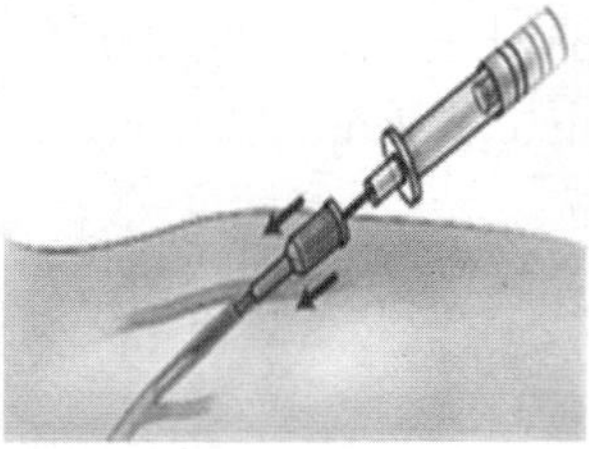

4.________________ 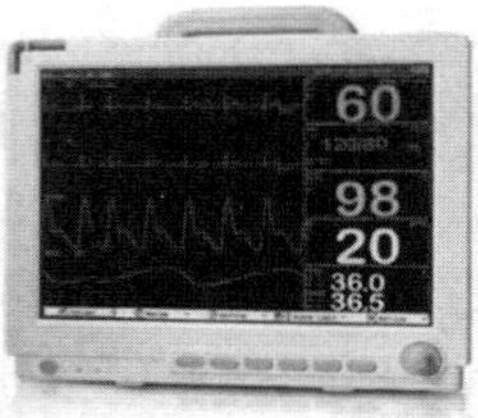 5.________________ 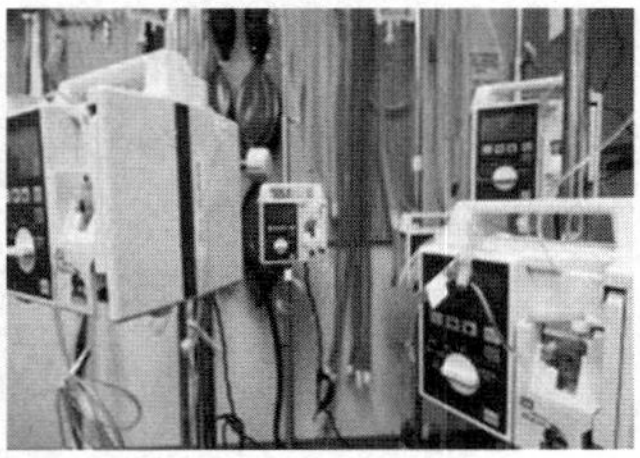 6.________________

Task 2: Warming-up

Directions: Watch the video clip from the movie *Awake* and try to answer the questions below. While watching the video, please take notes in the blanks to help you to follow the content.

1) What happened to the man in the video?

2) How did he feel being awake but paralyzed in the surgery?

Notes

Text B Awareness under TIVA[1]: A Doctor's Personal Experience

K.J. ROWAN

1. Awareness can be a **devastating** complication of anesthesia. I share my experience as a general practitioner[2], awake but paralyzed whilst undergoing a laparoscopic **cholecystectomy** under TIVA. I write this in the hope of preventing this from happening to others.

2. During my second pregnancy I suffered **recurrent bouts** of **biliary colic**. A laparoscopic cholecystectomy was planned at two months **postpartum**.

3. After placement of intravenous lines the anesthetist began administering the anesthetic. I complained of pain in my arm, so he then administered **lignocaine**, which partially relieved it. I then had a mask placed over my face. Shortly after this I felt light-headed and thought I might be starting to go off to sleep. Then suddenly I felt I could not breathe. I was totally alert. I could not feel my chest rising and I had no sensation of air moving in or out. It was

devastating /ˈdevəsteɪtɪŋ/ adj. 毁灭性的

cholecystectomy /ˌkɒlɪsɪsˈtektəmɪ/ n. 胆囊切除术

recurrent /rɪˈkʌrənt/ adj. 反复出现的

bout /baʊt/ n.（疾病的）发作

biliary colic /ˈbiljəri ˈkɔlik/ n. 胆绞痛

postpartum /ˌpəʊstˈpɑːtəm/ adj. 产后

lignocaine /ˈlɪgnəkeɪn/ n. 利诺卡因，二乙氨基（麻醉用）

a terrifying feeling. I attempted to scream but only a short yell came out and then I could no longer make a sound. My tongue felt as if it was stuck to the roof of my mouth. At the same time I tried to raise my hand to my chest to **notify** someone that I couldn't breathe. I felt it move a few inches and then it would no longer move. Someone beside me asked what was wrong but I could no longer respond. I went into a state of panic. I tried to **reassure** myself that the anesthetist would see my oxygen saturations[3] on the monitor and realize I couldn't breathe. I tried to move my whole body but could not move anything, not even my eyes which were now closed. It was a wrestle of my mind against the rest of my body. I felt like my mind was **thrashing** around inside my head every time I tried to move. The torture for my mind became too much and I eventually gave up the effort to move.

notify /ˈnəʊtɪfaɪ/ v. 通知

reassure /ˌriːəˈʃʊə(r)/ v. 使……安心

thrash /θræʃ/ v.（使）激烈扭动

4. I realized that I was not supposed to be awake at this stage and that the anesthetist and other medical staff in the operating theatre did not know. I waited for them to respond. I felt so alone.

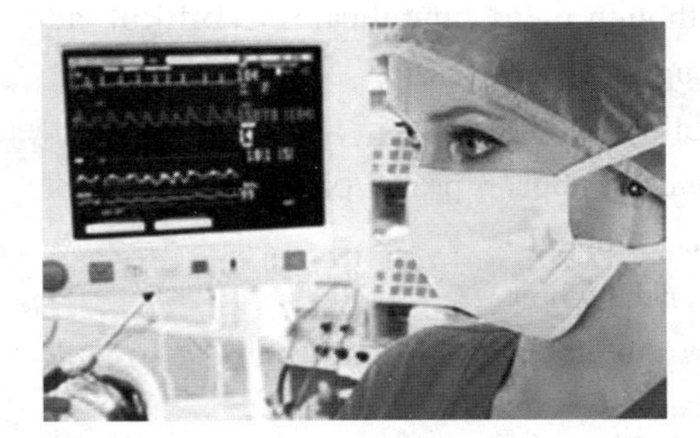

5. I was tachycardiac and sweating **profusely**. The anesthetic record confirmed this and showed

profusely /prəˈfjuːslɪ/ adv. 大量地

a rise in blood pressure from 110/70 to 185/125. I felt the tube going down my throat as I was **intubated**. I heard someone say I had gone into **bigeminy**. There appeared to be some alarm amongst the staff, I thought I was going to have a serious arrhythmia and they were about to get the paddles out to shock me.

intubate /ˈɪntjʊbeɪt/ v. 插管

bigeminy /baɪdˈʒemɪnɪ/ n. 二联律（如心脏的律动一跳是两下）

6. I could feel the cool **iodine** being sponged onto my abdomen. I was terrified as I realized I had sensation and was going to feel the surgery. I was not sure if it would be possible to survive through the pain of a whole operation. I prayed to God. My eyes were taped closed and the **drapes** were laid over my body including my face. I was extremely hot and felt as if I was suffocating. With my face now covered over I felt completely cut off from the medical staff. I heard the surgeon ask the anesthetist if he should go ahead and start surgery. I had a split second glimmer of hope as I thought maybe they had realized things were too abnormal to begin the surgery. When the anesthetist replied "yes", my heart sank. I could only lie and wait for the incision.

iodine /ˈaɪədiːn/ n. 碘

drape /dreɪp/ n. 消毒帷

7. The first **umbilical** incision, although only a few centimeters long felt like a huge incision across my abdomen. Even more painful was the pressure of the **probes** pushing around my upper abdomen. The pain went on and on. I thought I would have to lie there and bear it for the whole operation. The anesthetist withdrew the drapes from my face and lifted my eyelids on several occasions. I could see him looking down at me but I couldn't move my eyes. I longed for him

umbilical /ʌmˈbɪlɪkəl/ adj. 肚脐的

probe /prəʊb/ n. 医用探针

to see some sign that I was awake but he simply closed my eyelids again.

8. I am not sure how much longer after this I was awake. I was given **midazolam** and **opiates** which may have affected my recall of events. At some stage (about 20 to 30 minutes into the procedure) the problem was recognized and I was finally put to sleep.

midazolam /mɪdəzəʊ'læm/ n. 咪达唑仑

opiate /'əʊpɪət/ n. 麻醉剂

9. I woke up in the recovery room crying uncontrollably. I was told there was an anesthetic pump failure. I felt overwhelmingly **traumatized** by my experience but was also relieved to know that I had survived.

traumatize /'traʊməˌtaɪz/ v. 受精神创伤

10. On the ward following this, I was very **drowsy**. My eyes wanted to close and go to sleep but I wouldn't let them. Every time I started to drift off to sleep I would make myself wake up. I didn't want to lose control. A therapist visited me and my husband not long after the operation. I talked through all I remembered for the first time. Although this was painful, being able to share my experiences enabled me to feel a slight sense of relief.

drowsy /'draʊzi/ adj. 昏昏欲睡的

11. I felt so distressed that I didn't know if I would fully recover from this experience. The next few days were very hard. I had a lot of anxiety, and some nightmares. The experience was played over and over in my mind especially when I lay down in bed to try and sleep. I felt fear when I lay on my back and closed my eyes, but every day got a little better. For the next couple of weeks I was fearful of more accidents happening. I was anxious going out in the car and unusually fearful when I flew in an aeroplane a couple of weeks later.

12. Throughout this I tried to remain positive. I chose not to dwell on this experience but to move on into normal life as fast as possible. Even so I occasionally have mulled over the experience and still at times feel a little distressed.

13. I now know that this occurred because of the failure of a SIMS Graseby 3500 TCI pump[4] in administering a propofol total intravenous anesthetic. A discussion of the cause of this pump's failure has been recently published. I received a 5 ml **bolus** of propofol at the time of induction but none from that time until the point when the pump failure was recognized. The display on the Graseby pump indicated that a more than adequate dose of propofol was being delivered, however the **syringe** driver did not move, so no propofol was actually delivered. As blood concentrations of propofol cannot be measured intraoperatively there was no objective measure to show the absence of propofol in my blood. My clinical signs of tachycardia, bigeminy, hypertension and profuse sweating were present prior to the first skin incision. Unfortunately these signs were initially attributed to the surgical stimulus so there was a significant delay in recognizing the problem.

bolus /'bəʊləs/ n.（单次给药的）剂量

syringe /sɪ'rɪndʒ/ n. 注射器

14. I underwent surgery, paralyzed and awake. I had complete awareness and full sensation of pain. If I had been administered an inhalational agent[5], end-tidal gas[6] concentrations would have been measured and this complication would not have occurred. I do not wish other people to experience what I have, so I ask the question—why does the anesthetic profession use this method which cannot be objectively monitored? (1286 words)

Notes:

1. TIVA: 全称是 total intravenous anesthesia, 静脉内全麻醉
2. general practitioner: 全科医生，普通医师
3. oxygen saturation: 血氧饱和度
4. SIMS Graseby 3500 TCI pump: 英国 SIMS Graseby 公司生产的靶控输注泵
5. inhalational agent: 吸入性麻醉药
6. end-tidal gas: 终末潮气

While You Read

Task 1: Reading Skills Practice

Directions: Read the text very quickly and try to find out the invalid arguments made in the text (See ***Skills Bank***) Then, try to fill in the blanks with the invalid arguments made in the text and write down the style of the fallacy.

	Invalid Arguments	Style
1		Argument to the people
2		Argument to the person
3		Bandwagon Appeal
4		Red Herring

Task 2: Text-related Presentation

Directions: Read carefully the part of Text B that corresponds to your task, and prepare a 1-min presentation in a unique and creative way. Remember to turn in the slip with the details of your task to your teacher before you present. (The slip can be found at the end of the book)

1) Explain to the class what TIVA is. (Para.1)

2) Introduce the concept of awareness under anesthesia and explain how it happens. (Para.1)

3) Tell in the tone of the author her emotional and physical change before the incision. (Para.3-Para.6)

4)Talk about the physical mental experience of the author during the procedure. (Para.7-Para.8)

5) Introduce the concept of post-trauma stress disorder(PTSD) based on the author's experience. (Para.4-Para.12)

6) Compare TIVA with inhalationed anesthesia and explain why the auther claimed inhalational agent was safer. (Para.14)

After You Read

Task 1: Oral Presenting

Directions: Try to rephrase or explain the following sentences without using the boldfaced words or phrases. (This is going to be integrated into the communicative interaction in the classroom. The task can be done orally in the classroom.)

1. General anesthesia is a drug-induced, **reversible** state of **unconsciousness**, loss of memory, pain relief and relaxation of muscles.
2. All intravenous drugs and anesthetic gases are **administered in appropriate amounts** so that the patient is completely unconscious during the surgery, but awake and pain free at the end.
3. The skin and tissues that the needle goes through are also numbed with local anesthetic so that there is **minimal discomfort** associated with placement of the needle.
4. **Accounts of** recall and helplessness while paralyzed have made unconsciousness **a primary concern** of patients **undergoing** general anesthesia.
5. I had **a split second glimmer of hope** as I thought maybe they had realized things were too abnormal to begin the surgery.

Task 2: Critical Thinking

Directions: Work in groups and discuss the following questions. At the end of your discussion, each group will assign a representative to present your pints on this issue.

For various reasons, patients may suffer from anesthetic awareness during surgery which can lead to post-traumatic stress disorder, a severe anxiety disorder that can arise after a terrifying ordeal. How can doctors avoid the tragedy? If it is inevitable, how can doctors help patients alleviate post-traumatic anxiety?

After-class Tasks

Task 1: Collocations

Directions: Complete the following word chunks taken from Text A and Text B according to their Chinese equivalents and make a sentence with each word chunk.

1. ________ anesthesia 全身麻醉
2. ________ anesthesia 局部麻醉
3. ________ of memory 失忆
4. ________ state 可逆状态
5. muscle________ 肌松剂
6. ________ injection 静脉注射
7. ________ tube 呼吸管
8. ________ anesthetic 喷雾式麻醉药
9. nerve ________ 神经阻滞
10. ________ 剖腹产
11. ________ 全科医生
12. ________ the anesthetic 注射麻醉药
13. oxygen ________ 血氧饱和
14. anesthetic ________ 麻醉泵
15. syringe ________ 注射器
16. ________ sweating 大量出汗
17. ________ dose 充足的剂量
18. ________ colic 胆绞痛
19. second ________ 二次怀孕
20. anesthetic pump ________ 麻醉泵故障

Task 2: Translation

Directions: Translate sentence 1 to 3 into Chinese and pay close attention to the translation of the words in bold. Then translate sentence 4 to 6 into English using the words in the bracket.

1. At the end of the operation, the effect of the muscle relaxants is **reversed with** two other drugs, and the anesthetic gases discontinued.

   ____

   ____

2. All intravenous drugs and anesthetic gases are **administered in appropriate amounts** so that the patient is completely unconscious during the surgery, but awake and pain free at the end.

   ____

   ____

3. My clinical signs of tachycardia, bigeminy, hypertension and profuse sweating were present **prior to** the first skin incision.

   ____

   ____

4. 他总是想着麻醉苏醒后所经历过的种种恐怖。(dwell on)

____

____

5. 最新医学研究证实了健康生活方式的好处。(confirm)

____

____

6. 他们开始从痛苦的梦魇中慢慢恢复过来。(recover from)

____

____

Task 3: Listening & Speaking

Directions: Watch the video and complete the guided note-taking.

Word Bank

obese /əʊˈbiːs/ ad. 肥胖的	vital signs 生命体征
blood clots 血块	pressure cuffs 血压袖带
body mass index (BMI) 身体质量指数	diabetes /ˌdaɪəˈbiːtiːz/ n. 糖尿病
obstructive /əbˈstrʌkˌtɪv/ ad. 阻塞性的	apnea 呼吸暂停
windpipe /ˈwɪndpaɪp/ n. 气管	endotracheal tube 气管内管

1. ______________________________
- difficult to monitor ________________
- take a longer time to ________________
- high risk for ________, ________, ________.
- difficult to obtain ________________
- hard to introduce ________________
- challenging ____________ control

2. Obesity and its related illnesses

BMI: ____________

Illnesses related to obesity include: ______________

Task 4: Research

Directions: Do some research into the *life of an anesthesiologist in China.* You can introduce the work and life of an anesthesiologist and explain to us why Chinese anesthesiologists are more vulnerable to sudden death. You can present in the form of an interview, short play or simply a lecture. Make sure each member of the group will present his or her part on the stage.

Resources

http://journals.lww.com/anesthesia-analgesia/pages/default.aspx
http://www.nlm.nih.gov/medlineplus/anesthesia.html

Task 5: Writing

Directions: Anesthesia is considered to be the most humane and merciful of all of mankind's accomplishments in that it relieves the pain and suffering of human beings. With the popularity of anesthesia technology, mankind begins their journey to seek more comfort in whatever way they can. The pain that used to be bearable is unacceptable today without anesthesia. Is anesthesia reducing people's tolerance for pain? Is it a good blessing or a curse in disguise? Please illustrate your point.

Task 6: Vocabulary Log

Directions: Please finish the vocabulary log (Please find the log at the end of the book) by looking up the dictionary and write down the words or expressions you have learnt in this unit by following the examples already listed in the log. And then write down the translation for each vocabulary item and if possible, its variants, synonym, antonym and the frequent collocations.

Task 7: Reading Log

Directions: After learning the whole unit and conducting the research, you have known more about anesthesia from different perspectives. You can go to the library or surf on the internet for more knowledge about it. You can take down the key information according to the sample chart. (Please find the chart at the end of the book)Also you are allowed to complete the chart on a computer or tablet so that this section is expandable if you want to write more than the space on a paper form might allow. And then send it to your teacher by emails. The reading log can serve as an informal way to keep track of your reading progress.

Unit 8

Administration of Drugs

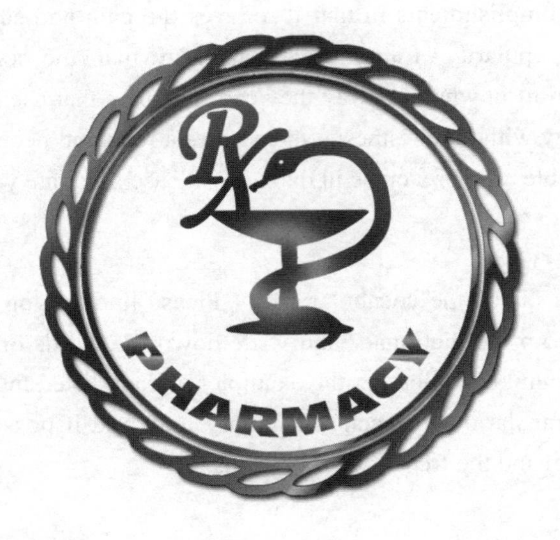

Only about seventy years ago was chemistry, like a grain of seed from a ripe fruit, separated from the other physical sciences. With Black,Cavendish and Priestley, its new era began. Medicine, pharmacy, and the useful arts, had prepared the soil upon which this seed was to germinate and to flourish.

——Justus von Liebig

Skills Bank

Decoding the Text's Structure

Every text has a structure. Understanding the text structure will help you understand what the writer is trying to do. Usually, the title can indicate what type of essay it is. And the type of the essay can help readers to predict its structure. No matter which kind of essay it is, it usually includes the following parts:

The introduction.

It may be general statements about the subject. The purpose is to provide background and to attract readers' attention. It may include definitions of key terms in the text. It should also include statement of the specific subdivisions of the topic and/or indication of how the topic is going to be tackled. It should introduce the central idea or the main purpose of the writing.

The main body.

The main body consists of one or more paragraphs of ideas and arguments. Each paragraph develops a subdivision of the topic. The paragraphs of the essay contain the main ideas and arguments of the essay together with illustrations or examples. The paragraphs are linked in order to connect the ideas. The purpose of the essay must be made clear and the reader must be able to follow its development.

The conclusion.

The conclusion includes the writer's final points. It should recall the issues raised in the introduction and draw together the points made in the main body and explain the overall significance of the conclusions. It should clearly signal to the reader that the essay is finished and leave a clear impression that the purpose of the essay has been achieved.

Pre-class Tasks

Task 1: Medical Terminology Study

Directions: Study the word roots, prefixes and suffixes listed in the table below and do the **Vocabulary Preview** exercise for Text A or/ and Text B according to your teacher's instructions.

Roots	Meaning
pharmac/o	drug 药物
crani/o	skull 颅
immun/o	immune 免疫
neur/o	nerve 神经
nephr/o	kidney 肾
terat/o	monster; malformed fetus 畸形
adren/o	adrenal gland 肾上腺
limph/o	lymph 淋巴
Prefixes	**Meaning**
intra-	within 内，内部
anti-	against 反，对抗，抑制，退，代替
Suffixes	**Meaning**
-pathy	disease 病
-logy	study ……学
-gen	substance that produces ……原

Task 2: Prepared Individual Presentation

Directions: The assigned students need to prepare a 1-min oral presentation concerning the questions in **Text-related Presentation** for Text A and/or Text B as required by your teacher.

Task 3: The Muddiest Points

Directions: Read Text A and Text B in the study group to find out the sentences that are the least clear to you after your discussions, the viewpoints that you disagree with and the understanding you have achieved through discussions and the questions you want to put forward concerning the content of the texts. Put the above information in a slip and send it to the teacher via WeChat 24 hours prior to the class. (The slip can be found on the last page of the book.)

In-class Tasks

Text A

Before You Read

Task 1: Vocabulary Preview

Directions: Divide the following words into their word parts and then give their Chinese translations based on the table above.

Medical Terms	Prefix	Word Root(s)	Suffix	Chinese
pharmacological				
intracranial				
immunological				
neuroleptic				
nephropathy				
carcinogenesis				
adrenocortical				
antiplatelet				
antigen				
lymphocyte				
antibiotics				
myeloma				

Task 2: Warming-up

Directions: Watch the video carefully and try to answer the questions below. While watching the video, please take some notes in the blanks to help you to memorize the information.

1) According to the video, what are the consequences of adverse drug reactions?

2) Why are the elderly more vulnerable to adverse reactions?

Notes

Text A Adverse Drug Reactions

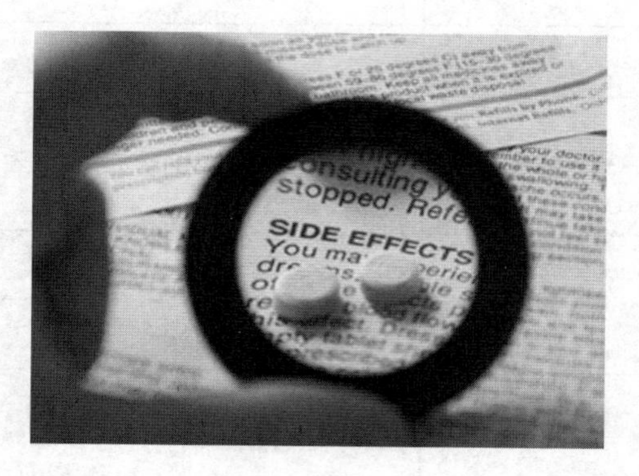

1. Adverse drug reactions are unwanted effects caused by normal **therapeutic** doses[1]. Drugs are great **mimics** of disease, and adverse drug reactions present with diverse clinical signs and symptoms. The classification proposed by Rawlins and Thompson divides reactions into type A and type B.

therapeutic /ˌθerəˈpjuːtɪk/ adj. 治疗（学）的；疗法的

mimic /ˈmɪmɪk/ n. 模仿

2. Type A reactions, which constitute **approximately** 80% of adverse drug reactions, are usually a consequence of the drug's primary **pharmacological** effect (e.g. bleeding from warfarin[2]) or a low therapeutic index (e.g. nausea from digoxin[3]), and they are

approximately /əˈprɒksɪmətli/ adv. 大约

pharmacological /ˌfɑːməkəˈlɒdʒɪkl/ adj. 药学的

therefore predictable. They are dose-related and usually mild, although they may be serious or even fatal (e.g. **intracranial** bleeding from warfarin). Such reactions are usually due to inappropriate dosage, especially when drug elimination is **impaired**. The term "side effects" is often applied to minor type A reactions.

intracranial /ˌɪntrəˈkreɪnɪəl/ adj. 颅内的

impair /ɪmˈpeə(r)/ v. 损害，削弱

3. Type B ("**idiosyncratic**") reactions are not predictable from the drug's main pharmacological action, are not dose-related and are severe, with a considerable mortality. The underlying **pathophysiology** of type B reactions is poorly if at all understood, and often has a genetic or immunological basis. Type B reactions occur infrequently (1:1000--1:10,000 treated subjects being typical).

idiosyncratic /ˌɪdɪəsɪŋˈkrætɪk/ adj. 怪异的

pathophysiology /ˈpæθəʊfɪzɪˈɒlədʒɪ/ n. 病理生理学

4. Three further minor categories of adverse drug reaction have been proposed:

type C – continuous reactions due to long-term drug use (e.g. neuroleptic-related tardive dyskinesia[4] or analgesic nephropathy[5]);

type D – delayed reactions (e.g. alkylating agents[6] leading to **carcinogenesis**, or retinoid-associated teratogenesis[7]);

type E – end-of-use reactions, such as **adrenocortical** insufficiency following withdrawal of glucocorticosteroids[8], or withdrawal syndromes following discontinuation of treatment with benzodiazepines[9] or β-adrenoceptor antagonists[10].

carcinogenesis /kɑːsɪnəʊˈdʒenɪsɪs/ n. 癌变

adrenocortical /əˌdriːnəʊˈkɔːtɪkəl/ adj. 肾上腺皮质的

5. In the UK there are between 30,000 and 40,000 medicinal products available directly or on **prescription**. Surveys suggest that

prescription /prɪˈskrɪpʃn/ n. 药方；处方

approximately 80% of adults take some kind of medication during any two-week period. Exposure to drugs in the population is thus substantial, and the incidence of adverse reactions must be viewed in this context. Type A reactions are reported to be responsible for 2–3% of consultations in general practice. In a recent prospective analysis of 18,820 hospital admissions by Pirmohamed et al. (2004), 1,225 were related to an adverse drug reaction (prevalence 6.8%), with the adverse drug reaction leading directly to admission in 80% of cases. Median bed stay was eight days, accounting for 4% of hospital bed capacity. The projected annual cost to the NHS[11] is £466 million. Overall fatality was 0.15%. Most reactions were either definitely or probably avoidable. Adverse drug reactions are most frequent and severe in the elderly, in **neonates**, women, patients with hepatic or renal impairment, and individuals with a history of previous adverse drug reactions. Such reactions often occur early in therapy (during the first one to ten days). Drugs most commonly **implicated** include low-dose aspirin (anti-platelet agents), diuretics, warfarin and NSAIDs[12]. A systematic review by Howard et al. (2006) of preventable adverse drug reactions which caused hospitalization, implicated the same major drug classes.

neonate /ˈniːəʊneɪt/ n. 新生儿

implicate /ˈɪmplɪkeɪt/ v. 密切关联

6. It is often difficult to decide whether a clinical event is drug related, and even when this is probable, it may be difficult to

determine which drug is responsible, as patients are often taking multiple drugs. One or more of several possible approaches may be appropriate.

7. A careful drug history is essential. The following considerations should be made to assess **causality** of the effect to the drug: did the clinical event and the time course of its development fit with the **duration** of suspected drug treatment and known adverse drug effects? Did the adverse effect reverse upon drug withdrawal and, upon re-challenge with the drug, reappear? Were other possible causes reasonably excluded? A patient's drug history may not always be conclusive because, although **allergy** to a drug implies previous exposure, the **antigen** may have occurred in foods (e.g. **antibiotics** are often fed to livestock and drug residues remain in the flesh), in drug mixtures or in some casual manner.

8. **Provocation** testing. This involves giving a very small amount of the suspected drug and seeing whether a reaction ensues, e.g. skin testing, where a drug is applied as a patch, or is pricked or scratched into the skin or injected **intradermally**. Unfortunately, **prick** and scratch testing is less useful for assessing the systemic reaction to drugs than it is for the more usual **atopic** antigens (e.g. pollens), and both false-positive and false-negative results can occur. Patch testing is safe, and is useful for the diagnosis of contact **sensitivity**, but does not reflect systemic reactions and may

causality /kɔːˈzælətɪ/ n. 因果关系

duration /djuˈreɪʃn/ n. 持续时间

allergy /ˈælədʒɪ/ n. 过敏

antigen/ˈæntɪdʒən/ n. 抗原

antibiotics /ˌæntɪbaɪˈɒtɪks/ n. 抗生素

provocation /ˌprɒvəˈkeɪʃn/ n. 诱发

intradermally /ˌintəˈdəːməli/ adv. 皮内注射的

prick /prɪk/ v. 刺，扎

atopic /eɪˈtɒpɪk/ adj. 异位的

sensitivity /ˌsensəˈtɪvətɪ/ n. 灵敏性

itself cause allergy. Provocation tests should only be undertaken under expert guidance, after obtaining informed **consent**, and with **resuscitation** facilities available.

consent /kən'sent/ v. 同意；赞成
resuscitation /rɪˌsʌsɪ'teɪʃn/ n. 恢复知觉

9. **Serological** testing and lymphocytes testing. Serological testing is rarely helpful, circulating antibodies to the drug do not mean that they are necessarily the cause of the symptoms. The demonstration of transformation occurring when the patient's lymphocytes are exposed to a drug ex vivo suggests that the patient's T-lymphocytes are **sensitized** to the drug. In this type of reaction, the **hapten** itself will often provoke lymphocyte transformation, as well as the **conjugate**.

serological /sɪrə'lɒdʒɪkəl/ adj. 血清学的
sensitize /'sensətaɪz/ v. 活化；强化
hapten /'hæpten/ v. 半抗原
conjugate /'kɒndʒəgeɪt/ n. 结合物

10. The best approach in patients on multiple drug therapy is to stop all potentially causal drugs and reintroduce them one by one until the drug at fault is discovered. This should only be done if the reaction is not serious, or if the drug is essential and no chemically unrelated alternative is available. All drug allergies should be recorded in the case notes and the patient informed of the risks involved in taking the drug again. (906 words)

Notes:

1. therapeutic doses: 治疗剂量
2. warfarin: 华法林抗凝血素，又名灭鼠灵
3. Digoxin: 地高辛，一种强心药，被广泛用于治疗心脏病
4. tardive dyskinesia: 迟发性运动障碍
5. analgesic nephropathy: 镇痛剂肾病，是因长期服用镇痛药物而引起的慢性肾炎
6. alkylating agents: 烷化剂，一种抗肿瘤药

7. retinoid-associated teratogenesis: 维甲酸相关的致畸作用
8. withdrawal of glucocorticosteroids: 停用糖皮质激素
9. Benzodiazepines: 苯环类药物，精神类药物
10. β-adrenoceptor antagonists: 肾上腺素受体拮抗剂
11. NHS: 全称为 National Health Service，英国国家医疗服务系统
12. NSAIDs: 全称为 non-steroidal anti-inflammatory drugs，非类固醇抗炎药

While You Read

Task: Text-related Presentation

Directions:Take turns to make a 1-min presentation about the following topics. Your presentation should be based on the text but not limited to the text. You are encouraged to present in a unique and creative way.

1) Give a detailed explanation to type A reaction. (Para. 2)

2) What are the main characteristics of type B reaction? (Para. 3)

3) Can you use concrete examples to tell us the key information about type C、D and E reaction? (Para. 4)

4) What are the proper approaches to deal with the adverse drug reactions? (Para.6-Para.10)

After You Read

Task 1: Academic English Study

Directions: Read this section carefully and try to find examples of hedging from Text A and Text B.

Hedging

It is often believed that academic writing, particularly scientific writing, is factual, simply to convey facts and information. However it is now recognized that an important feature of academic writing is the concept of cautious language, often called “hedging” or “vague language”. In other words, it is necessary to make decisions about your stance on a particular subject, or the strength of the claims you are making. Different subjects prefer to do this in different ways.

Language used in hedging:

1.	Introductory verbs	e.g. seem, tend, appear to be, think, believe, doubt, be sure, indicate, suggest
2.	Certain lexical verbs	e.g. believe, assume, suggest
3.	Certain modal verbs	e.g. will, must, would, may, might, could
4.	Adverbs of frequency	e.g. often, sometimes, usually
5.	Modal adverbs	e.g. certainly, definitely, clearly, probably, possibly, perhaps, conceivably,
6.	Modal adjectives	e.g. certain, definite, clear, probable, possible
7.	Modal nouns	e.g. assumption, possibility, probability
8.	That clauses	e.g. It could be the case that. / It might be suggested that.
9.	To-clause + adjective	e.g. It may be possible to obtain. / It is important to develop.

For example:

1) Surveys ***suggest*** that ***approximately*** 80% of adults take some kind of medication during any two-week period.

2) The following considerations ***should*** be made to assess causality of the effect to the drug.

3) Such reactions are ***usually*** due to inappropriate dosage, especially when drug elimination is impaired.

Task 2: Critical Thinking

Directions: Work in groups and discuss the following questions. At the end of your discussion, each group will assign a representative to present your opinions on this issue.

A newspaper headline goes that **"Drug-makers Abandon Nature's Pharmacy"**. *From penicillin to Taxol, most new drugs have had their roots in natural products, but scientists worry that the approach is in decline.*

What do you think of the reasons behind? What are your opinions about this? Or do you have any better ideas for its solution? You may use specific examples to support your ideas.

Text B

Before You Read

Task 1: Vocabulary Preview

Directions: Preview the words in the table below and use them to describe the following pictures.

fetus myeloma obstetrician leprosy phocomelia depression

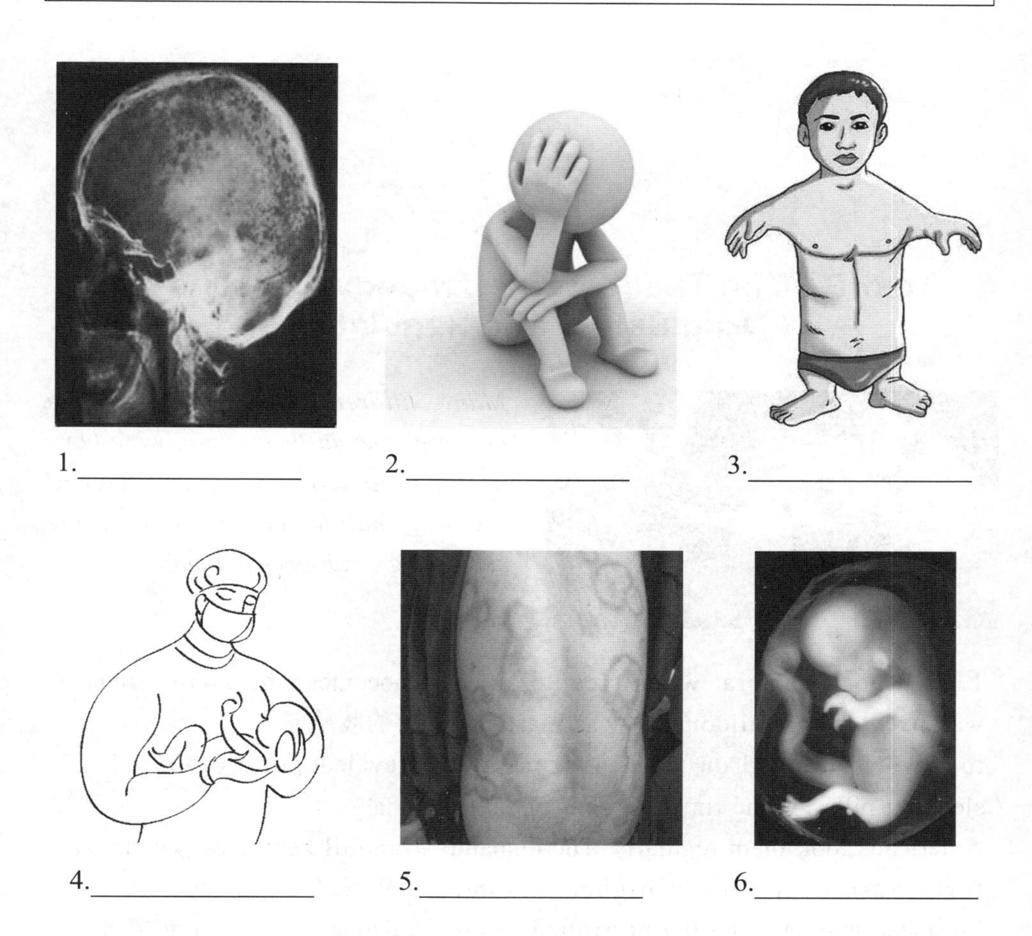

1.________________ 2.________________ 3.________________

4.________________ 5.________________ 6.________________

Task 2: Warming-up

Directions: Watch the video carefully and try to answer the questions below. While watching the video, please take some notes in the blank to help you to memorize the information.

1) What is the video about?

2) According to the video, what would happen to the babies after women took this drug during their pregnancy?

Notes

Text B The Thalidomide Tragedy: Lessons for Drug Safety and Regulation

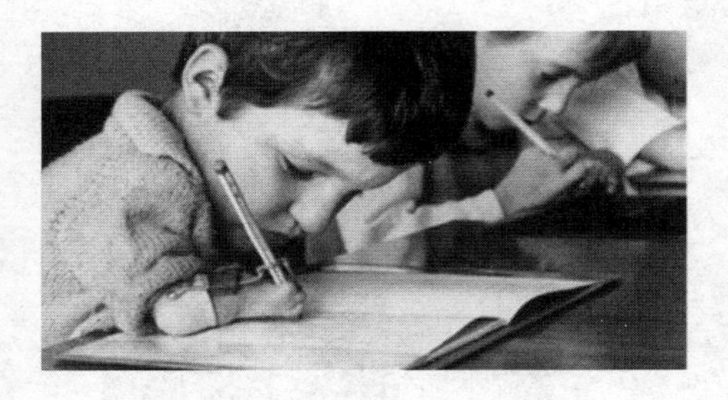

*Many children in the 1960's, like the kindergartner in the picture, were born with **phocomelia** as a side effect of the drug thalidomide, resulting in the shortening or absence of limbs.*

1. In a post-war era[1] when sleeplessness was **prevalent**, thalidomide[2] was marketed to a world hooked on **tranquilizers** and sleeping pills. At the time, one out of seven Americans took them regularly. The demand for **sedatives** was even higher in some European markets, and the **presumed** safety of thalidomide, the only non-barbiturate sedative[3] known at the time, gave the drug massive appeal. Sadly, tragedy followed its release, **catalyzing** the beginnings of the rigorous drug approval and monitoring systems in place at the United States Food and Administration (FDA)[4] today.

phocomelia /fəʊkə'miːlɪə/ n. 海豹肢畸形

prevalent /'prevələnt/ adj. 流行的

tranquilizer /'træŋkwɪlaɪzə/ n. 镇静剂

sedative /'sedətɪv/ n. 镇静剂

presume /prɪ'zju:m/ v. 假定

catalyze /'kætəlaɪz/ v. 催化，促进

2. Thalidomide first entered the German market in 1957 as an over-the-counter remedy, based on the maker's safety claims. They advertised their product as "completely safe" for everyone, including mother and child, "even during pregnancy," as its developers "could not find a dose high enough to kill a rat." By 1960, thalidomide was marketed in 46 countries, with sales nearly matching those of aspirin.

3. Around this time, Australian **obstetrician** Dr. William McBride discovered that the drug also **alleviated** morning sickness. He started recommending this off-label use of the drug to his pregnant patients, setting a worldwide trend. Prescribing drugs for off-label purposes, or purposes other than those for which the drug was approved, is still a common practice in many countries today, including the U.S. In many cases, these off-label **prescriptions** are very effective, such as prescribing **depression** medication to treat **chronic** pain.

obstetrician/ˌɒbstəˈtrɪʃn/ n. 产科医师

alleviate /əˈliːvɪeɪt/ v. 减轻，缓和

prescription /prɪˈskrɪpʃn/ n. 处方

depression/dɪˈpreʃn/ n. 抑郁，沮丧

chronic /ˈkrɒnɪk/ adj. 慢性的

4. However, this practice can also lead to a more prevalent **occurrence** of unanticipated, and often serious, adverse drug reactions. In 1961, McBride began to associate this so-called harmless **compound** with severe birth defects in the babies he delivered. The drug interfered with the babies' normal development, causing many of them to be born with phocomelia, resulting in shortened, absent, or flipper-like limbs. A German newspaper soon reported 161 babies were adversely affected by thalidomide, leading the makers of the drug—who had ignored reports of the birth defects associated

occurrence /əˈkʌrəns/ n. 发生

compound /ˈkɒmpaʊnd/ n. 化合物

with it—to finally stop distribution within Germany. Other countries followed suit and, by March of 1962, the drug was banned in most countries where it was previously sold.

5. In July of 1962, president John F. Kennedy[5] and the American press began praising their **heroine**, FDA inspector Frances Kelsey[6], who prevented the drug's approval within the United States despite pressure from the **pharmaceutical** company and FDA supervisors. Kelsey felt the application for thalidomide contained incomplete and insufficient data on its safety and effectiveness. Among her concerns was the lack of data indicating whether the drug could cross the **placenta**, which provides **nourishment** to a developing **fetus**.

heroine /'herəʊɪn/ n. 女英雄

pharmaceutical /ˌfaːmə'suːtikl/ adj. 药学的，药物的

placenta /plə'sentə/ n. 胎盘

nourishment /'nʌrɪʃmənt/ n. 营养物，滋养物

fetus /'fiːtəs/ n. 胚胎，胎儿

6. She was also concerned that there were not yet any results available from U.S. clinical trials of the drug. Even if these data were available, however, they may not have been entirely reliable. At the time, clinical trials did not require FDA approval, nor were they subject to **oversight**. The "clinical trials of thalidomide involved distributing more than two and a half million tablets of thalidomide to approximately 20,000 patients across the nation—approximately 3,760 women of childbearing age, at least 207 of whom were pregnant. More than one thousand physicians participated in these trials, but few tracked their patients after **dispensing** the drug.

oversight /'əʊvəsaɪt/ n. 疏忽，失察

dispense /dɪ'spens/ v. 配药

7. The tragedy surrounding thalidomide and Kelsey's wise refusal to approve the drug helped

motivate profound changes in the FDA. By passing the Kefauver-Harris Drug **Amendments** Act[7] in 1962, **legislators** tightened restrictions surrounding the **surveillance** and approval process for drugs to be sold in the U.S., requiring that manufacturers prove they are both safe and effective before they are marketed. Now, drug approval can take between eight and twelve years, involving animal testing and tightly regulated human clinical trials.

amendment /ə'mendmənt/ n. 修正

legislator /'ledʒɪsleɪtə(r)/ n. 立法委员；立法者

surveillance /sɜː'veɪləns/ n. 监督；监测

8. Despite its harmful side effects, thalidomide is FDA-approved for two uses today—the treatment of inflammation associated with Hansen's disease (**leprosy**) and as a chemotherapeutic agent for patients with multiple **myeloma**, purposes for which it was originally prescribed off-label. Because of its known adverse effects on fetal development, the dispensing of thalidomide is regulated by the System for Thalidomide Education and Prescribing Safety (S.T.E.P.S.) program. The S.T.E.P.S. program, designed by Celgene pharmaceuticals and carried out in pharmacies where thalidomide prescriptions are filled, educates all patients who receive thalidomide about potential risks associated with the drug.

leprosy /'leprəsi/ n. 麻风病

myeloma /ˌmaɪə'ləumə/ n. 骨髓瘤

9. Thalidomide has also been associated with a higher occurrence of blood clots and nerve and blood disorders. Northwestern University's **pharmacovigiliance** team, Research on Adverse Drug Events And Reports (RADAR), has launched a joint project with the Walgreens pharmacy[8] at Northwestern Memorial Hospital

pharmacovigiliance /fɑːməkʌ'vɪdʒɪləns/ n. 药物警戒性

so that these side effects may be understood and monitored, like those affecting fetal development. RADAR, led by Dr. Charles Bennett of the Feinberg School of Medicine, combines the expertise of clinicians, academics, pharmacists, and statisticians to monitor and **disseminate** information about adverse drug reactions to cancer drugs

disseminate /dɪ'semɪneɪt/ v. 散布，传播

10. Their project tracks the number of patients who get a blood clot after receiving thalidomide, whether or not the patient received an **anticoagulant** drug, which are used to help prevent clotting, and if so, which drug was used. Tracking this information will help researchers better identify the incidence and prevention of thalidomide-associated blood clots, allowing the drug to continue to serve as an effective therapy for many patients. (891words)

anticoagulant /ˌæntikəʊ'ægjələnt/ n. 抗凝剂

Notes:

1. Thalidomide: 沙利度胺，是德国制药商格兰泰公司20世纪50年代推出的一种镇静剂，因其对减轻妇女怀孕早期出现的恶心、呕吐等反应有效，所以又名反应停。
2. In a post-war era: 战后时期，特指第二次世界大战结束之后的一段时期。
3. non-barbiturate sedative: 非巴比妥类的镇静剂
4. United States Food and Drug Administration (FDA) : 美国食品药品监督局，是国际医疗审核权威机构，由美国国会即联邦政府授权，是专门从事食品与药品管理的最高执法机关。
5. John F. Kennedy: 美国第35任总统，美国著名的肯尼迪家族成员，美国历史上最年轻的当选总统。1963年11月22日在达拉斯遇刺身亡。
6. Frances Kelsey: 美国FDA医学官员，顶住各方压力坚持不通过沙利度胺在美国上市，避免了沙利度胺悲剧在美国的危害，因此获得了总统颁发的联邦公务人员特别奖，之后还列入了美国国家妇女名人堂。

7. Kefauver-Harris Drug Amendments Act:1962 年美国国会通过的《Kefauver-Harris 药品修正案》以保证药品功效和更好的药品安全性。
8. the Walgreens pharmacy: 世界 500 强企业之一沃尔格林药房，是仅次于美国 CVS 连锁药房的第二大全国药房连锁店。

While You Read

Task 1: Reading Skills Practice

Directions: Read the title of the text and write down your predication of what the author is going to write about and how the contents are going to be structured. Then read the text quickly to finish the structure table with the help of the skills above. (See ***Skills Bank***)

Your Predication

1. What type of essay will it be?
2. What will the author talk about in the essay?
3. How will these aspects be structured?

Structure

	Main Idea	Supporting Details	Paragraph
Introduction	Thalidomide entered the market as an OTC remedy.	1. Thalidomide was marketed to a world hooked on tranquilizers and sleeping pills. 2. 3.	Para 1-3
Main body	Thalidomide led to a more prevalent occurrence of unanticipated, and often serious, adverse drug reactions.	1. McBride began to associate thalidomide with severe birth defects in the babies he delivered. 2. 3.	Para 4-6
Conclusion	How the tragedy drew more attention to the drug safety.	1. 2.	Para7- 10

Task 2: Text-related Presentation

Directions:Read carefully the part of Text B that corresponds to your task, and prepare a 1-min presentation in a unique and creative way. Remember to turn in the slip with the details of your task to your teacher before you present. (The slip can be found at the end of the book)

1) Introduce the drug thalidomide to the class (Para.1)
2) Explain the concept of over-the-counter medicine (Para.2)
3) Explain the off-label use of drugs (Para.3)
4) Explain the definition and the different stages of clinical trial (Para.6)
5) Explain the procedures of drug approval (Para.7-Para.9)
6) Tell us about Frances Kelsey and the setbacks she experienced to prevent the Thalidomide tragedy

After You Read

Task 1: Oral Presenting

Directions: Try to rephrase or explain the following sentences without using the boldfaced words or phrases. This is going to be integrated into the communicative interaction in the classroom. The task can be done orally in the classroom.

1. The demand for sedatives was even higher in some European markets, and **the presumed safety of thalidomide**, the only non-barbiturate sedative known at the time, **gave the drug massive appeal**.
2. They advertised their product as "completely safe" for everyone, including mother and child, "even during pregnancy," as its developers "**could not find a dose high enough to kill a rat.**"
3. In many cases, **these off-label prescriptions** are very effective, such as prescribing depression medication to treat chronic pain.
4. A German newspaper soon reported 161 babies were **adversely affected by thalidomide**, leading the makers of the drug who had ignored reports of the birth defects associated with it **to finally stop distribution** within Germany.
5. Among her concerns was the lack of data indicating **whether the drug could cross the placenta**, which provides nourishment to a developing fetus.

Task 2: Critical Thinking

Directions: Work in groups and discuss the following questions. At the end of your discussion, each group will make a list of your key points in a table and select a reporter to present your opinions. The group members should take turns to report and take notes in this semester.

1) What can we learn from the thalidomide tragedy?

2) What are the effective ways to ensure the drug safety and effectiveness?

After-class Tasks

Task 1: Word Chunks

Directions: Complete the following word chunks taken from Text A and Text B according to their Chinese equivalents and make a sentence with each word chunk.

1. ________ drug reactions 药物不良反应
2. therapeutic ________ 治疗剂量
3. clinical ________ 临床症状
4. ________ effect 副作用
5. ________ action 药理作用
6. ________ product 医药产品
7. on ________ 凭处方
8. hospital ________ 入院
9. drug ________ 用药史
10. __________ testing 激发试验
11. ________ testing 血清学检测
12. sleeping ________ 安眠药
13. non-barbiturate ________ 非巴比妥类镇静药
14. ________ morning sickness 缓解晨吐
15. ________ pain 慢性疼痛
16. birth ________ 出生缺陷
17. ________ the babies' normal development 阻碍婴儿正常发育
18. ________ suit 如法炮制
19. clinical ________ 临床试验
20. drug ________ 药品批准

Task 2: Translation

Directions: Translate sentence 1 to 3 into Chinese and pay close attention to the translation of the words in bold. Then translate sentence 4 to 6 into English using the words in the bracket.

1. Sadly, **tragedy followed its release**, **catalyzing the beginnings of** the rigorous drug approval and monitoring systems in place at the United States Food and Drug Administration (FDA) today.

____

____

2. **Prescribing drugs for off-label purposes**, or purposes other than those for which the drug was approved, is still **a common practice** in many countries today, including the U.S.

____

____

3. The drug **interfered with** the babies' **normal development**, causing many of them to be born with phocomelia, **resulting in** shortened, absent, or flipper-like limbs.

____

____

4. 她认为，有关反应停应用的安全性和有效性数据还不够完整和充足。(application)

____

____

5. 当时临床试验不需要经过 FDA 的许可，也缺乏监管。(subject to)

____

____

6. 反应停还会引起血栓和神经及血液紊乱。(occurrence)

____

____

Task 3: Listening & Speaking

Directions: Watch the video and take down notes under the clues listed below before you make an oral summary of what have heard from the video.

Word Bank

dosage /ˈdəʊsɪdʒ/ n. 剂量　　transdermal /tˈrænzdɜːməl/ adj. 经皮吸收的

By definition, prescription compounding is preparing medication for a single patient based on their individual prescription, not making large bulk quantities for stock. Some examples of compounding application include:

- patients ________________ such as a very small dose for a child.
- Patients ________________ such as turning a pill to a liquid or transdermal gel for patients who can not swallow pills.
- Patients ________________, such as one without gluten or colored dyes.
- Patients ________________ because of low profitability.
- Patients ________________
- ________________ including flavored medicated treats or even ear gels that carry medication through the skin to avoid the difficulty of administering oral medications.

Task 4: Research

Directions: Do some research into How Drugs are Developed and Approved in the United States in the Past Twenty Years. Discuss and exchange ideas within your group to have an outline of the whole process. Then brainstorm on the following aspects in groups before you develop your discussions into an oral presentation for the next class. You can present in the form of an interview, short play or simply a lecture. Make sure each member of the group will present his or her part on the stage.

1) What is the mission of U.S. Food and Drug Administration (FDA)?
2) How are drugs developed?
3) How can a new drug product be introduced to the market?
4) How can FDA ensure that drugs marketed in this country are safe and effective?

Resources

Here are the websites where you can find the useful information for your research.
http://www.registrarcorp.com/?gclid=CNrcre-J_b8CFcMJvAoddGYAnQ
http://www.fda.gov/

Task 5: Writing

Directions: *Text B gives us an account of the Thalidomide tragedy happening around the world.* In the pharmaceutical history, there were many other infamous tragedies caused by the adverse reactions of the drugs. Please do some research on the internet to gather information about the most influential pharmaceutical tragedies in history and choose one to write a narrative titled the ***Ups and Downs of*** ________.

Task 6: Vocabulary Log

Directions: Please finish the vocabulary log (Please find the log at the end of the book) by looking up the dictionary and write down the words or expressions you have learnt in this unit by following the examples already listed in the log. And then write down the translation for each vocabulary item and if possible, its variants, synonym, antonym and the frequent collocations.

Task 7: Reading Log

Directions: After learning the whole unit and conducting the research, you have known more about drug approval and drug safety from different perspectives. You can go to the library or surf on the internet for more knowledge about it. You can take down the key information according to the sample chart. (Please find the chart at the end of the book.) Also you are allowed to complete the chart on a computer or tablet so that this section is expandable if you want to write more than the space on a paper form might allow. And then send it to your teacher by emails. The reading log can serve as an informal way to keep track of your reading progress.

Unit 9

Healing Power of TCM

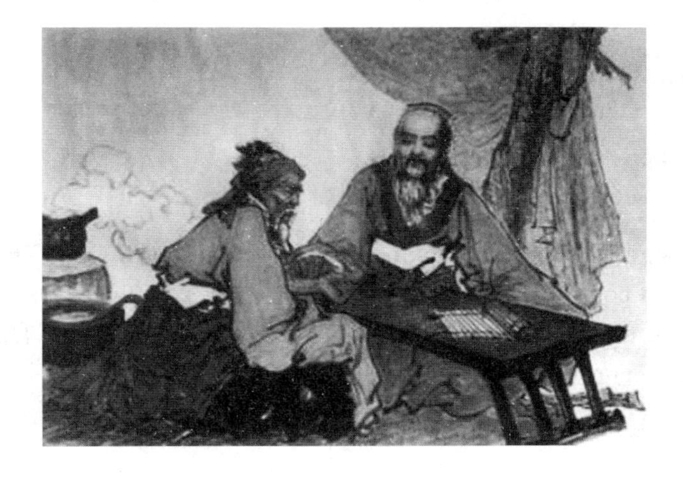

Only the healing art enables one to make a name for himself and at the same time give benefit to others.

——Chinese Proverb

Skills Bank

Detecting Writing Purpose

Finding the purpose in a passage is closely related to finding the main idea. The main idea of a passage reflects the author's purpose in writing the passage. By identifying the main idea, you will be better able to distinguish between those purposes that are found in the passage and those that are not. More than one purpose may be present in a passage.

There are four Purpose Categories:

1. To inform
2. To persuade
3. To narrate
4. To describe

1. To inform

These passages attempt to teach or explain something to you. The passage will explain a point, a certain process, or a concept. Usually, when a passage's purpose is to inform, you will find objective language and facts. The passage should not contain opinions or bias language.

2. To persuade

These passages attempt to convince the reader, to argue a position, or to prove a point. In this type of passage, authors are trying to get your support for their position or belief. They want you to agree with them and will word their passages accordingly.

Since the purpose is to persuade you, the passages usually contain a mixture of facts and opinions.

3. To narrate

These passages recount a sequence of events or tell a story to the reader. The events in the passage may be either fact or fiction. Since the author is telling you about an event or about a series of events, most of these passages are in some form of time order.

4. To describe

These passages make some appeal to your five senses: hearing, sight, smell, touch, or taste. In these passages, you will often be given information that will form a picture or an image of the topics discussed. When passages are written to describe something, they contain information about the physical properties or the characteristics of the "something" they are describing.

Pre-class Tasks

Task 1: Medical Terminology Study

Directions: Study the word roots, prefix and suffix listed in the table below and do the **Vocabulary Preview** exercise for Text A or/ and Text B according to your teacher's instructions.

Roots	Meaning
path/o	disease 疾病
gnos/o	knowledge 知识
pharmac/o	drug, medication 药，药物，药学
somn/o	sleep 睡觉
gynec/o	woman 女性，女子
men/o	menses; menstruation 与月经有关的
acu/	needle; sharp 针；尖锐
cardi/o	heart 心，心脏
orph/o	啡
morph/o	form, shape 形态，形
Prefix	**Meaning**
dia-	through, during, across 通过，透析，横
neo-	new 新
hetero-	the other (of two), another; different 其他；异；不同
in-	not 不，非，否定
pro-	before; forward 先；前进
peri-	surrounding, around 周，近，围绕
endo-	inside, within 内
Suffix	**Meaning**
-osis	a process or state, disease or increase 过程或状态，病，病态

续表

Suffix	Meaning
-logy	the study of……学；……论
-gen	to be born; of a certain kind 发生；原
-ic	pertaining to 属于……的，有……特性的
-ia	condition 情况，状况，状态
-logist	someone who studies a certain field; a specialist 研究者；学家
-um	structure; tissue; thing 结构；组织；东西
-in	a substance, chemical, chemical compound 素，质
-ine	a substance, chemical, chemical compound 生物碱，素，有机碱

Task 2: Prepared Individual Presentation

Directions: The assigned students need to prepare a 1-min oral presentation concerning the questions in **Text-related Presentation** for Text A and/or Text B as required by your teacher.

Task 3: The Muddiest Points

Directions: Read Text A and Text B in the study group to find out the sentences that are the least clear to you after your discussions, the viewpoints that you disagree with and the understanding you have achieved through discussions and the questions you want to put forward concerning the content of the texts. Put the above information in a slip and send it to the teacher via WeChat 24 hours prior to the class. (The slip can be found on the last page of the book.)

In-Class Tasks

Text A

Before You Read

Task 1: Vocabulary Preview

Directions: Divide the following words into their word parts and then give their Chinese translations based on the table above.

Medical Terms	Prefix	Word Root(s)	Suffix	Chinese
pathology				
diagnosis				
pharmacology				
heterogeneous				
pathogenic				
insomnia				
gynecologist				
menopause				
prognosis				
pericardium				
endorphin				

Task 2: Warming-up

Directions: Watch the video carefully and try to answer the questions below. While watching the video, please take some notes in the blanks to help you to memorize the information.

1) What does ancient Chinese philosophy hold?

2) According to the video, what is the theory of yin and yang?

3) What are the five elements or phases? How do they describe the visceral functions?

4) What is the unique theory of TCM?

Notes

Text A Traditional Chinese Medicine

1. Systematic reviews show that Chinese herbs and **acupuncture** can be effective for **atopic eczema** and chemotherapy-induced nausea, respectively. Traditional Chinese Medicine (TCM) is one of the oldest healing systems. TCM includes herbal medicine[1], acupuncture, **moxibustion**, massage, food therapy, and physical exercise, such as shadow boxing[2]. TCM is a fully **institutionalized** part of Chinese health care and widely used with western medicine. In 2006, the TCM sector provided care for over 200 million outpatients and some 7 million inpatients, accounting for 10%–20% of health care in China.

acupuncture /'ækjupʌŋktʃə(r)/ n. 针灸
atopic /eɪ'tɒpɪk/ adj. 特（异反）应性
eczema/'eksɪmə/ n. 湿疹
moxibustion /ˌmɒksɪ'bʌstʃən/ n. 艾灸
institutionalize /ˌɪnstə'tjuːʃənlaɪz/ vt. 制度化

2. Most of the principles of TCM were derived from the philosophical basis that contributed to the development of **Taoism**, and **Confucianism**. Ancient Chinese scholars noted that all natural phenomena could be **categorized** into Yin and Yang (two opposite, complementary, interdependent, and exchangeable aspects of nature), everything in the universe consisted of five basic elements (wood, fire, earth, metal, and water[3]), and the universe was constantly changing towards dynamic balance or harmony. Such knowledge was applied to understand, prevent, and cure disease.

Taoism /'taʊɪzəm/ n. 道教
Confucianism /kən'fjuːʃənɪzm/ n. 孔教，儒教
categorize ['kætəgəraɪz] v. 归类

3. In TCM, Yin refers largely to the material aspects of the organism and Yang to functions. There is a circulation of Qi (energy) and blood[4].

The organs work together by regulating and preserving Qi and blood through the so-called channels and **collaterals**[5]. Disease occurs after a disturbance in Yin–Yang or flow of Qi or blood, or disharmony in the organs caused by **pathogenic** (eg, sadness, joy, lifestyle) and climatic factors (dampness, heat, cold). Treatment aims to expel or suppress the cause and restore balance.

collateral /kəˈlætərəl/ n. 络

pathogenic /ˈpæθəˈdʒenɪk/ adj. 病原的，致病的

4. Imbalance is assessed by four traditional examination methods: looking, listening and smelling, asking, and touching[6]. Observations of the pulse, face, tongue, urine, and stool provide essential information. The diagnosis is derived with theories such as the eight **diagnostic** principles to differentiate between Yin–Yang, exterior–interior, deficiency–excess, and cold–heat, the five elements theory to assess the relations between organs and functions, and the **visceral manifestation** theory[7] to establish the disease location.

diagnostic /ˌdaɪəgˈnɒstɪk/ adj. 诊断的

visceral /ˈvɪsərəl/ adj. 内脏的

manifestation /ˌmænɪfeˈsteɪʃn/ n. 表示，显示

5. The diagnosis that guides treatment is called Zheng[8], a temporary state at one time and which is like a syndrome defined by symptoms and signs. The same disease in western medicine can manifest in different Zhengs and vice versa. Thus, treatment in the same patient varies over time and the same disease can be treated differently. For example, kidney Yin deficiency as a Zheng has three components: kidney, Yin, and deficiency. Other examples include **preponderant** liver Yang, flaring up of heart fire, and spleen–stomach dampness–heat. For each or a combination of the

preponderant /prɪˈpɒndərənt/ adj. 占有优势的

components, there are specific herbs or treatments. For example, bitter herbs are cool in nature and can be used to treat heat-ridden diseases[9]. TCM can make diagnoses and treat patients without needing a scientific understanding of cause and **pathogenesis**.

pathogenesis /ˌpæθəˈdʒenɪsɪs/ n. 发病机制

6. Acupuncture was introduced in developed countries in the 1600s. **Variolation** was developed in the 16th century in China as a method to immunise people against smallpox. Dried smallpox scabs were blown into the nose of an individual who then developed a mild form of the disease and lifelong resistance. The method was introduced to Europe in the early 1700s. **Artemisinin** and **ephedrine** are also derived from Chinese herbs.

variolation /vəraɪəˈleɪʃn/ n. 接种

artemisinin /ɑːtɪˈmɪsɪn/ n. 蒿素

ephedrine /ˈefɪdriːn/ n. 盐酸麻黄素

7. TCM was challenged by western medicine in China in the late 19th century. Western medicine had its most notable effects in surgery and public health, areas that had not been well developed in China until then. The increasing emphasis on western medicine **slackened** the development of TCM in the early 20th century. Since 1949, TCM has been scientifically studied and integrated with western medicine. Biomedical sciences have made considerable changes to TCM. For example, standardized formula of herbal therapies are now commonly used as tablets, capsules, and even **ampoules** as well as the traditional **decoctions** of individualized prescriptions.

slacken /ˈslækən/ vt.& vi.（使）放慢；（使）放松

ampoule /ˈæmpuːl/ n. 一次用量的针剂，安瓿

decoction /dɪˈkɒkʃən/ n. 煎药

8. The **integration** of TCM and western medicine[10] has been widely promoted and studied in China. Integration aims to eventually combine the two systems. Currently, integration is mainly at the level of physicians who have received training and can treat patients in both. For example, over a third of the training in TCM schools is in western medicine, and western-medicine schools also offer some training in TCM.

integration /ˌɪntɪ'greɪʃn/ n. 结合

9. Despite decades of research and integration, the fundamentals of TCM remain largely unchanged and its theories **inexplicable** to science.The absence of scientific understanding has caused **skepticism** and criticism about TCM. However, randomized trials[11] have shown efficacy for some TCM therapies.The efficacy of most assessed therapies, however, remains uncertain, often because of the low methodological quality of trials. Furthermore, most of these trials are published in Chinese, inaccessible to western doctors, and not included in systematic reviews. Selective publication of positive trials is another problem. The quality of TCM trials could be improved by adopting the bias-reduction points in the CONSORT[12] guidelines. Meanwhile, the patient, intervention, **comparator**, and outcome should also be carefully documented. For example, it is important to compare TCM with a **placebo** or an intervention of proven efficacy rather than interventions with unknown effects. Furthermore, patients' inclusion

inexplicable /ˌɪnɪk'splɪkəbl/ adj. 无法解释的

skepticism /'skeptɪsɪzəm/ n. 怀疑论，怀疑主义

comparator /'kɒmpəreɪtə/ n. 比较仪

placebo /plə'siːbəʊ/ n. 安慰剂

and exclusion criteria, and indications and contraindications of the tested therapy, must be specified clearly in a language comprehensible to users who have never learnt TCM. Tested herbal products also need to be standardized to ensure manufacturing consistency. **Standardization** is similarly important for diagnosis and procedural treatments, such as acupuncture. (892 words)

standardization /stændədaɪˈzeɪʃn/ n. 标准化

Notes:

1. herbal medicine: 中草药
2. shadow boxing: 太极拳
3. five basic elements: 五行，金木水火土
4. Qi and blood: 气血
5. channels and collaterals: 经络
6. looking, listening and smelling, asking, and touching: 中医四诊：望闻问切
7. visceral manifestation theory: 脏象理论
8. Zheng:（中医诊断）症
9. heat-ridden diseases: 热症
10. the integration of TCM and western medicine: 中西医结合
11. randomized trials: 随机试验
12. CONSORT: 全称为 Consohdated Standards of Reporting Trials，20 世纪 90 年代中期，国际上一个由临床流行病学家、临床专业人员、统计学家和医学杂志编辑组成的课题组，花费近 2 年的时间制作了一个随机对照临床试验报告的规范，并在国际著名的临床医学杂志上应用。实践应用规范的结果表明，临床试验报告的质量有了很大提高。这一报告规范称为"CONSORT 声明"。

While You Read

Task: Text-related Presentation

Directions: Take turns to make a 1-min presentation on the following topics. Your presentation should be based on the text but not limited to the text. You are encouraged to present in a unique and creative way.

1) Describe the coverage of TCM by giving examples. (Para. 1)

2) Give explanations on the Yin-Yang doctrine and Five-element theory? (Para. 2-4)

3) What is Zheng in TCM? Give some examples to explain it. (Para. 5)

4) Can you make use of concrete examples to illustrate the healing power of acupuncture?(Para. 6)

5) What is your opinion on the advantages and disadvantages of TCM? (Para. 9)

After You Read

Task 1: Academic English Study

Directions:Read this section carefully and find examples of precision language from Text A and Text B.

Precision

In academic writing you need to be precise when you use information, dates or figures. Do not use "a lot of people" when you can say "50 million people".

For example:

1. In **2006**, the TCM sector provided care for over **200 million** outpatients and some **7 million** inpatients, accounting for **10%–20%** of health care in China. (Para. 1)
2. The diagnosis is derived with theories such as the **eight** diagnostic principles to differentiate between Yin–Yang, exterior–interior, deficiency–excess, and cold–heat, the **five** elements theory to assess the relations between organs and functions, and the visceral manifestation theory to establish the disease location. (Para. 4)

Task 2: Critical Thinking

Directions: Work in groups and discuss the following questions. At the end of your discussion, each group will assign a representative to present your opinions on this issue.

Sometimes TCM is combined with western medicine to conduct treatment. Many people think it is the western medicine that really works. What's your opinion about it? According to the text, we know that the integration of TCM and western medicine has been widely promoted and studied in China. Do you think western medicine and Chinese traditional medicine can coexist in a harmonious condition? Is it possible that Chinese traditional medicine will eventually lose its importance?

Text B

Before You Read

Task 1: Vocabulary Preview

Directions: Preview the words in the table below and use them to describe the following pictures.

insomnia	gynecologist	menopause
acupuncture	pericardium	pharmacology

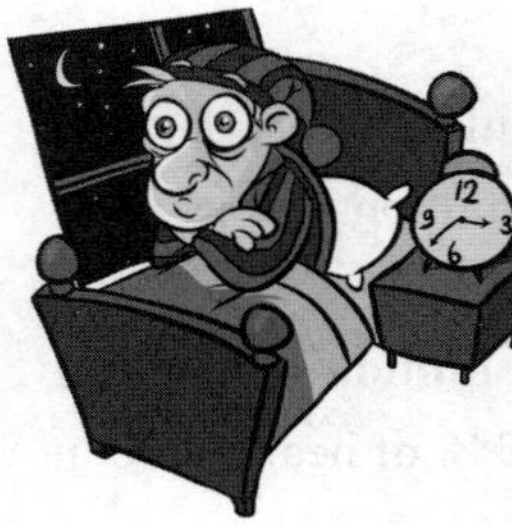

1. 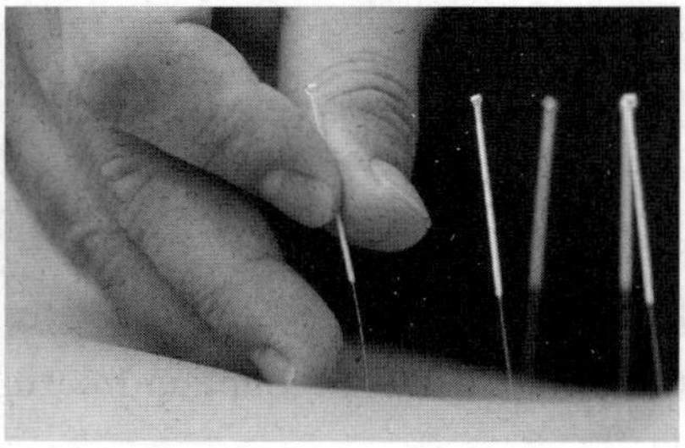 ________________ 2. 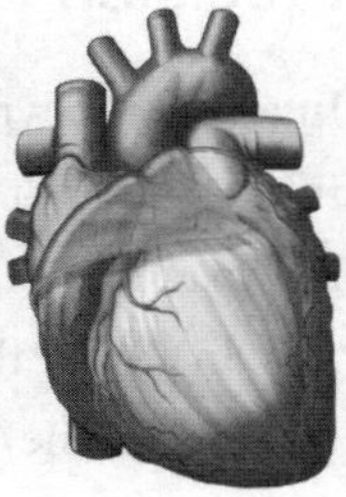 ________________ 3. ________________

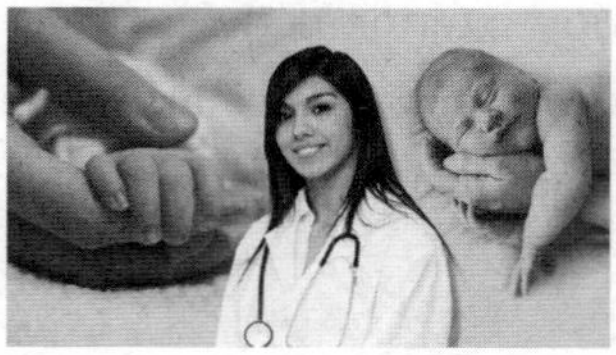

4. 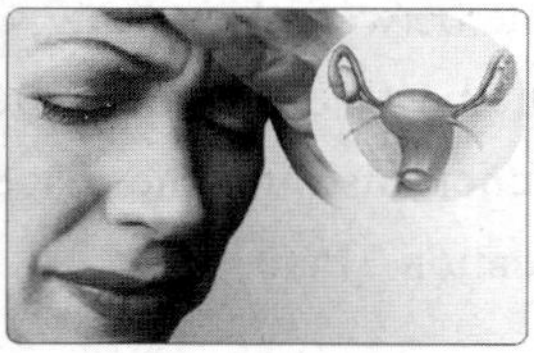 ________________ 5. 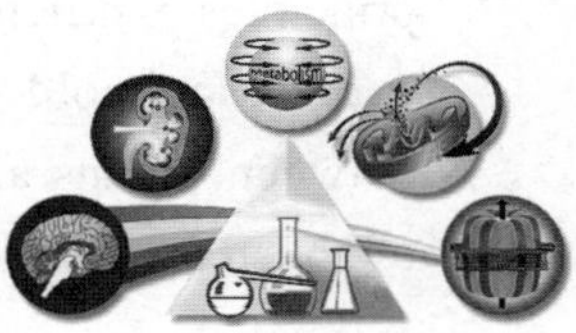 ________________ 6. ________________

Task 2: Warming-up

Directions: Watch the video carefully and try to answer the questions below. While watching the video, please take some notes in the blanks to help you to memorize the information.

1) There is a variety of traditional Chinese therapy, what are mentioned in this video

clip?

2) What diseases and disorders can be treated by acupuncture?

3) What are the 15 manipulations in Tui-na therapy?

Notes

Text B Chinese Medicine in Action: Case Studies

1. The great doctor John H. Shen always reminded his students, "Disease is rooted in the life of the patient." Thus, the correct diagnosis is based on understanding the life of the patient. It is not limited to immediate symptoms. Each practitioner may assess the patient differently and come to **dissimilar** conclusions. Just as many roads lead to a destination, varied Chinese medicine approaches may lead to the same resolution to the "disease".

dissimilar /dɪˈsɪmɪlə/ adj. 不同的

2. Diagnosing Olga

3. The following case study is an example of how my particular diagnostic process works, drawing from several theories and weaving them together to form a diagnosis. I do not claim that my method is superior to that of other professionals. Rather, it shows how I

think in my daily practice, and provides a glimpse of how Chinese Medicine practitioners process patient information.

4. Olga, a single, forty-five-year-old preschool teacher, came for relief of **insomnia** and fatigue. Questioning revealed that she had more trouble staying asleep than falling asleep, and when she awakened, she noticed feeling warm. She often felt **irritable**, and was short-tempered[1] with her coworkers and the children in her care. She attributed[2] this to lack of sleep. Her **gynecologist** had diagnosed early **menopause** and had prescribed **hormone** therapy.

5. During our consultation, she revealed that she was often thirsty, and felt exhausted each morning, even on the rare occasions when she slept well. She also complained of [3]occasional lower back pain that had persisted over many years. She emitted a distinctly sour odor, had a gray-green facial tone, and **flushed** while speaking. Her voice was **monotone**. Her tongue tip was red, the tongue body pale, and the coating slightly greenish. Her pulse felt fast and weak, especially in the kidney position, where it was very deep, requiring strong pressure to feel it.

6. My most vivid observation was the sour odor and the green **tint** of her **complexion** and tongue; I therefore suspected a **disharmony** of the wood element, which corresponds to[4] the color green as well as to the liver organ. Treating the liver was obvious, but the question was how. There are many different

insomnia /ɪn'sɒmnɪə/ n. 失眠

irritable /'ɪrɪtəb(ə)l/ adj. 急躁的，易怒的

gynecologist /ˌgaɪnɪ'kɒlədʒɪst/ n. 妇科医生

menopause /'menəpɔːz/ n. 更年期

hormone /'hɔːməʊn/ n. 激素

flush /flʌʃ/ v. 脸红

monotone /'mɒnətəʊn/ adj. 单调的

tint /tɪnt/ n. 色彩

complexion /kəm'plekʃ(ə)n/ n. 肤色

disharmony /dɪs'hɑːmənɪ/ n. 不调和

Chinese medicine treatments for the liver. Using common terminology, practitioners can sooth the liver[5] , **dredge** the liver[6], nourish the liver[7], or cool the liver[8]. The exact nature of the treatment is **discerned** by looking deeper. The theory of Five Phases helps explain the nature of the distress. According to these principles, the kidney is mother to the liver, preceding it in the generating cycle. When the liver is in distress, look first at the kidney as the source. Noting Olga's chronic lower back pain and deep kidney pulse, I diagnosed the kidney as the likely source of disharmony, and realized it must be adjusted before an effective treatment of the liver would work.

dredge /dredʒ/ v. 疏浚

discern /dɪ'sɜːn/ v. 识别

7. According to the Five Phases theory[9], wood generates fire; therefore, the liver is mother to the heart. It also predicts that heart-related symptoms could appear if the liver is out of balance. In Olga's case, this had already happened, judging by her insomnia, **irritability**, and red-tipped tongue.

irritability /ˌɪrɪtə'bɪlɪtɪ/ n. 易怒

8. My treatment plan started to take shape. I knew that it must **encompass** at least three elements: water (kidney), wood (liver), and fire (heart). I knew with certainty that I must assist Olga to restore harmony, balance, and **normalcy** to these three organs. Whatever the nature of the distress, normalcy is the cure. Body imbalances, no matter how chemically complex, can be expressed symbolically as yin and yang. The theory of yin and yang **illuminates** the nature of this imbalance. Restoring balance depends on discerning yin

encompass /ɪn'kʌmpəs; en-/ vt. 包含，环绕

normalcy /'nɔrmlsi/ n. 常态

illuminate /ɪ'l(j)uːmɪneɪt/ v. 阐明

from yang and knowing which is in excess and which is deficient. When yin and yang are in proper balance, normalcy follows. All Chinese medicine practitioners evaluate their patients in terms of yin and yang, doing their best to determine what is in excess and what is deficient. Once this is completed, a treatment plan is apparent. This evaluation is based on what stands out or is prominent in the appearance, **demeanor**, behavior, and history of the individual.

demeanor /di'miːnə/ n. 举止

9. The Theory of the Organs[10] reveals that the kidney is a great **repository** of Qi. Surplus Qi is stored there. Olga's weak lower back and fatigue indicate a deficiency of kidney energy. Her thirst, dry skin, and heat-disturbed sleep pointed to a deficiency of yin fluids. It appeared that Olga's kidney yin, which would normally generate her liver yin fluids and in turn cool her liver, had become deficient, thus failing to cool the liver sufficiently, causing the liver yang to heat up, rising to scorch the heart, resulting in symptoms of rapid pulse, insomnia, and irritability.

repository /rɪ'pɒzɪt(ə)rɪ/ n. 仓库

10. In Chinese medicine terminology, my working diagnosis was "deficient kidney yin generates deficient liver yin causing excess yang of the liver and heart." My treatment plan became clear. To restore balance, I needed to assist Olga to strengthen the deficient yin fluids of both her liver and kidney and to reduce the excess yang fire in her liver and heart.

11. Armed with a working diagnosis, I then developed a treatment strategy. Having a plan provides perspective, guidance, and focus. Such a plan should **prognosticate** the length of time needed for symptomatic relief as well as complete resolution. The treatment plan should evaluate all available options, such as massage, movement, **meditation**, particular acupuncture points[11], and specific **herbal formulas**[12].

12. Since Olga had experienced sleep problems for five years, I anticipated approximately five months of treatment to affect a cure. But many of my patients feel better within days. I find most people with insomnia experience some relief after one or two acupuncture treatments or within a week of taking herbs.

13. I planned to put Olga on an acupuncture and herb **regimen**, but first suggested something else. From her voice, I suspected she felt dulled or depressed, so I recommended that she try to add something new to her life. As she reclined on her back on the acupuncture table, we discussed Tai Chi, yoga, and writing classes. But after I tapped a small needle in her third-eye point, yintang, her body relaxed and her eyes closed. I placed thin needles in the insides of her wrists in the heart and **pericardium** channels. **Endorphins** seeped like morphine into her bloodstream; soon she was asleep.

14. After thirty minutes, Olga woke up, forgetting at first where she was. I jokingly

prognosticate /prɒgˈnɒstɪkeɪt/ v. 预言

meditation /medɪˈteɪʃ(ə)n/ n. 冥想

herbal /ˈhɜːb(ə)l/ adj. 草药的

formula /ˈfɔːmjʊlə/ n. 配方

regimen /ˈredʒɪmən/ n. 养生法

pericardium /ˌperɪˈkɑːdɪəm/ n. 心包；心包膜

endorphin /enˈdɔːfɪn/ n. 内啡肽

morphine /ˈmɔːfiːn/ n. 吗啡

congratulated her on surviving her first acupuncture treatment. She said it was the best sleep she had experienced in years. I described her first herbal prescription, a combination of two popular formulas: shui de an, known for its ability to calm the spirit and clear heat from the heart, plus zhi bai di huang, to strengthen yin, and nourish the body's cooling and **lubricating** fluids.

lubricate /ˈlu:brɪkeɪt/ v. 润滑

15. Olga was practitioner's dream, a rare model patient who responds to all treatment by the book. After about six months of herbs and acupuncture, she was fundamentally cured. I see her now and then for minor **ailments**, but not for chronic insomnia or fatigue.

ailment /ˈeɪlm(ə)nt/ n. 疾病

16. I wish all my patients were like Olga, but I must claim: "Your mileage may vary." Most people experience noticeable relief, and acute, simple problems are often resolved immediately. Difficult problems are usually difficult for everybody, including practitioners of Traditional Chinese Medicine.

Notes:

1. be short-tempered with: 容易对……发脾气
2. attribute ...to...: 归咎于
3. complain of : 主诉
4. correspond to: 对应于
5. sooth the liver: (中医术语)平肝
6. dredge the liver: (中医术语)疏肝
7. nourish the liver: (中医术语)养肝
8. cool the liver: (中医术语)清肝
9. the Five Phases theory: 五行理论。它是将古代哲学理论中以木、火、土、金、水五类特性及其生克制化规律来认识、解释自然的系统结构和方法论运用到中医学而建立的中医基本理论，用以解释人体内脏之间的相互关系、脏腑组织器官的属性、运动变化及人体与外界环境的关系。

10. The Theory of the Organs: 脏腑学说。它是通过观察人体外在现象、征象，来研究人体内在脏腑的生理功能、病理变化及其相互关系的学说。
11. acupuncture points: 穴位
12. herbal formulas: 中药药方

While You Read

Task 1: Reading Skills Practice

Directions: The main idea of a passage reflects the author's purpose in writing the passage. Generally speaking, there are four Purpose Categories (see ***Skills Bank***). Read critically the 16 paragraphs and make an analysis of their writing purposes.

	Purpose categories	Para.	Clues in the text
Writing purposes	to inform		
	to persuade		
	to narrate	Para. 4	Olga, a single, forty-five-year-old preschool teacher
	to describe		

Task 2: Text-related Presentation

Directions:Take turns to make a 1-min presentation about the following topics. Your presentation should be based on the text but not limited to the text. You are encouraged to present in a unique and creative way.

1) The patient was diagnosed with early menopause. Please find more information about menopause on the internet and tell if the patient fit the description of the diagnosis. (Para. 4)

2) The doctor suspected patient had a disharmony of the wood element. What does it mean? (Para. 6)

3) Explain the sentence "When yin and yang are in proper balance, normalcy follows." (Para. 8)

4) The author used endorphin (western medicine) to treat the patient's insomnia. How do you think of using endorphin? (Para. 13)
5) How do you understand the sentence "Your mileage may vary"? (Para. 16)

After You Read

Task 1: Oral Presenting

Directions: Try to rephrase or explain the following sentences without using the boldfaced words or phrases.(This is going to be integrated into the communicative interaction in the classroom. The task can be done orally in the classroom.)

1. Just as many roads lead to a destination, varied Chinese medicine approaches may **lead to the same resolution to the "disease."**
2. The following case study is an example of how my particular diagnostic process works, **drawing from** several theories and **weaving them together to** form a diagnosis.
3. Using common terminology, practitioners can **sooth the liver**, **dredge the liver**, **nourish the liver**, or **cool the liver**.
4. All Chinese medicine practitioners evaluate their patients **in terms of** yin and yang, doing their best to determine **what is in excess and what is deficient**.
5. It appeared that Olga's kidney yin, which would normally generate her liver yin fluids and in turn cool her liver, had **become deficient**, thus failing to cool the liver sufficiently, causing the liver yang to **heat up**, rising to scorch the heart, **resulting in symptoms of** rapid pulse, insomnia, and irritability.

Task 2: Critical Thinking

Directions: Work in groups and discuss the following question. At the end of your discussion, each group will make a list of your key points and select a reporter to present your opinions. The group members should take turns to report and take notes in this semester.

We know that the integration of TCM and western medicine has been widely promoted and studied in China. Do you think western medicine and Chinese Traditional Medicine can coexist in a harmonious condition?

After-class Tasks

Task 1: Word Chunks

Directions: Complete the following word chunks taken from Text A and Text B according to their Chinese equivalents and make a sentence with each word chunk.

1. Traditional ________中医
2. health ________保健
3. ________ and blood 气血
4. channels and ________经络
5. looking, listening and smelling, asking, and ________望闻问切
6. ________ manifestation 脏象
7. ________ health 公共卫生
8. ________ formula 标准化配方
9. ________ points 穴位
10. ________trials 随机试验
11. ________of TCM and western medicine 中西医结合
12. herbal ________中药药方
13. early ________提早绝经
14. ________ of 主诉
15. ________ theory 五行学说
16. ________ balance 恢复平衡
17. minor ________小病
18. ________ the liver 养肝
19. Theory of ________脏腑学说
20. ________ Yang 阳气不足

Task 2: Translation

Directions: Translate sentence 1 to 3 into Chinese and pay close attention to the translation of the words in bold. Then translate sentence 4 to 6 into English using the words in the bracket.

1. TCM includes **herbal medicine**, **acupuncture**, **moxibustion**, **massage**, food therapy, and physical exercise, such as shadow boxing.

____

____

2. The organs work together by regulating and preserving Qi and blood through the so-called **channels and collaterals**.

____

____

3. It appeared that Olga's kidney yin, which would normally **generate** her liver yin fluids and in turn cool her liver, had **become deficient**, thus failing to cool the liver sufficiently, causing the liver yang to heat up, rising to scorch the heart, **resulting in symptoms of** rapid pulse, insomnia,

and irritability.

____

____

4. 古代的中国学者认为所有的自然现象都可以归为阴阳两类。(be categorized into)

____

____

5. 病人主诉偶尔腰下部疼痛，这种情况已持续多年。(complain of)

____

____

6. 根据五行理论，木生火；因此，肝滋养心脏。(generate)

____

____

Task 3: Listening & Speaking

Directions: Watch the video and finish the guided note-taking before making an oral summary of what have learnt from the video.

Word Bank

underneath /ʌndəˈniːθ/ prep. 在……的下面
imbalance /ɪmˈbæl(ə)ns/ n. 不平衡；不安定 lethargy /ˈleθədʒɪ/ n. 昏睡；嗜眠（症）

1. Literal translation of yin and yang:

Yin: ____

Yang: ____

2. The qualities that yin and yang represent:

Yin: ____

Yang: ____

3. Imbalance of Yin and yang will affect health

Too much yin will lead to: ______________________________

Not enough yin will lead to: ______________________________

Too much yang will lead to: ______________________________

Not enough yang will lead to: ______________________________

Task 4: Research

Directions: Do some research about the Traditional Chinese Medicine and then brainstorm the following aspects in groups before you develop your discussions into an oral presentation for the next class. You can present in the form of an interview, short play or simply a lecture. Make sure each member of the group will present his or her part on the stage.

1) Who are the legendary figures of TCM? Please give detailed description of them.
2) What's the difference of diagnosis between western medicine and TCM?
3) What is herbal medicine? Is it always safe to use them?
4) What's the condition of TCM in foreign countries in recently years?

Resources

Here are the websites where you can find the useful information for your research.
http://en.wikipedia.org/wiki/History_of_traditional_Chinese_medicine#Regulations
http://www.topchinatravel.com/china-medical-tourism/traditional-chinese-medicine-history.htm
http://www.travelchinaguide.com/intro/medicine.htm

Task 5: Writing

Directions: Write an essay titled ***1000 years of Chinese Medicine.*** Make sure you fully understand the text before writing and make your own voice clear. Your writing should include the three sections: preliminary, main text and end matter.

Task 6: Vocabulary Log

Directions: Please finish the vocabulary log (Please find the log at the end of the book) by looking up the dictionary and write down the words or expressions you have learnt in this unit by following the examples already listed in the log. And then write down the translation for each vocabulary item and if possible, its variants, synonym, antonym and the frequent collocations.

Task 7: Reading Log

Directions: After learning the whole unit and conducting the research, you have known more about TCM from different perspectives. You can go to the library or surf on the internet for more knowledge about it. You can take down the key information according to the sample chart. (Please find the chart at the end of the book) Also you are allowed to complete the chart on a computer or tablet so that this section is expandable if you want to write more than the space on a paper form might allow. And then send it to your teacher by emails. The reading log can serve as an informal way to keep track of your reading progress.

Unit 10

Professionalism of Nursing Practice

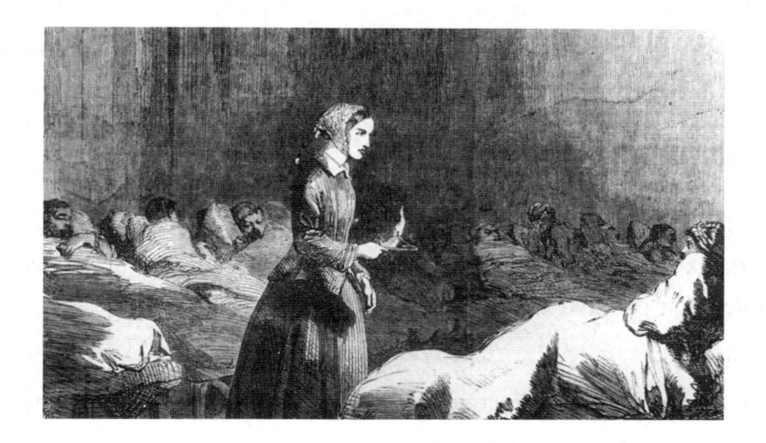

I will do all in my power to maintain and elevate the standard of my profession, and will hold in confidence all personal matters committed to my keeping and all family affairs coming to my knowledge in the practice of my calling.

With loyalty will I endeavor to aid the physician in his work, and devote myself to the welfare of those committed to my care.

——The Florence Nightingale Pledge

Skills Bank

Understanding the Author's Tone

The tone of a passage is the manner in which authors express their feelings or attitude about their topic. The author's tone is revealed through word choice and sentence structure.

There are two things you can look for when you are discerning the author's tone.

1. What type of words did the author use?

Remember, words have both denotative (dictionary definitions) and connotative (implications suggested above and beyond the dictionary definitions) meanings. Authors influence their readers by the words they choose to describe and discuss their topic.

2. What is the author's attitude about the topic?

Tone is strongly influenced by the author's attitude regarding the topic. If authors dislike their topic, their negative attitude will be evident. If authors like their topic, their positive attitude will be evident.

Tone Words

The following nouns and adjectives are commonly used to describe tone. This is not an all-inclusive list, but it is a good place to begin.

✧ abstruse absurd ambivalent amused
✧ angry apathetic arrogant awe
✧ bitter caustic cheerful comic
✧ compassionate complex condescending critical
✧ condemnation cruel cynical depressed
✧ detached distressed dignified disapproval
✧ earnest evasive excited farcical
✧ formal gentle ghoulish hard
✧ impassioned indignant intense
✧ intimate ironic irreverent joyous
✧ loving malicious mocking melancholy
✧ nostalgic objective optimistic
✧ outraged outspoken passionate pathetic

- ✧ pessimistic playful reticent reverent
- ✧ righteous sarcastic satirical sentimental
- ✧ serious scornful solemn sympathetic
- ✧ tragic uneasy unrealistic vindictive

Pre-class Tasks

Task 1: Medical Terminology Study

Directions: Study the word roots, prefixes and suffixes listed in the table below and do the **Vocabulary Preview** exercise for Text A or / and Text B according to your teacher's instructions.

Roots	Meaning
pneum/o	lungs 肺
tubercul/o	tuberculosis 结核病
arter/o	artery 动脉
tox/o	poison 毒
hem/o	blood 血
alb/o	white 白
sulph/o	containing sulphur 硫
bronch/o	the bronchi 支气管
Prefixes	**Meaning**
ex-	outward 外
poly-	multiple 多个
post-	after a particular date 之后 toward the spine in primates 背部
Suffixes	**Meaning**
-ia	a disease 病，症
-ory	of or relating to ……性质的，与……有关的
-osis	a process or state of a disease 病变状态
-escence	a process 变化，过程
-ation	a process or state 状态，过程
-ine	用以构成化学名词
-emia	blood 血
-globin	a colorless protein 蛋白

Task 2: Prepared Individual Presentation

Directions: The assigned students need to prepare a 1-min oral presentation concerning the questions in **Text-related Presentation** for Text A and / or Text B as required by your teacher.

Task 3: The Muddiest Points

Directions: Read Text A and Text B in the study group to find out the sentences that are the least clear to you after your discussions, the viewpoints that you disagree with and the understanding you have achieved through discussions and the questions you want to put forward concerning the content of the texts. Put the above information in a slip and send it to the teacher via WeChat 24 hours prior to the class. (The slip can be found on the last page of the book.)

In-class Tasks

Text A

Before You Read

Task: Warming-up

Directions: Watch the video "Nursing in China Sees Rapid Development" and try to answer the questions below. While watching the video, please take some notes in the blanks to help you to memorize the information.

1) What is the number of nurses in China by the end of 2010?

2) What's the ratio between doctors and nurses according to the video?

3) Where can we find nursing divisions?

Notes

Text A What's Nursing?

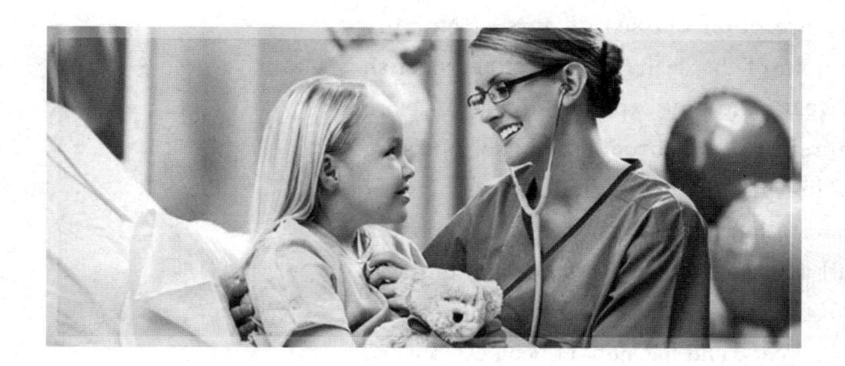

1. What is nursing? This may be a question in the mind of the young woman who is choosing a vocation. Usually, however, she is satisfied to think of nursing in terms of what she has seen or heard. A definition of nursing is probably of greatest interest to be the more thoughtful student or graduate nurse who is trying to see how she may increase her usefulness and at the same time distinguish her field of activity from[1] that of other groups of medical workers.

2. Presented here is not only the author's point of view but also the opinions of representative persons on such questions as: What is and what should be the function of the nurse? What **characterizes** the successful professional nurse, and what should be her preparation? It is important in discussing nursing activities, with which this text is chiefly concerned, to have arrived at some definite conclusions with relation to the nurse's responsibility or her place in the total program of medical care.

characterize /ˈkærəktəraɪz/ v. 具有……的特征

3. A definition of nursing cannot be confined to[2] the work of the professional nurse, because there are other classes of nurses. Nursing was born of the desire to protect and cherish the weak, and any expression of this desire is nursing in the broadest sense. Nursing is being practiced in some form wherever there are human beings, and it has existed in all ages; on the other hand, nursing as a profession is a product of approximately the last 75 years, and has not yet been established in all countries. William Osler[3], writing at the turn of the last century, called attention to the varied and enlarging functions of the nurse.

4. Nursing as an art to be **cultivated**, as a profession to be followed, is modern; nursing as a practice originated in the **dim** past, when some mother among the cave dwellers[4] cooled the forehead of her sick child with water from the brook, or first yielded to[5] the prompting to leave a well-covered bone and a handful of meal by the side of a wounded man left in the hurried flight before an enemy.

cultivate /ˈkʌltɪveɪt/ v. 培养

dim /dɪm/ adj. 暗淡的

5. As the needs of humanity change, with different times and conditions, out of the same **impulse** to serve, nursing has developed broader interests and functions. So we find in the dictionary that nursing has a wide range of meanings, which, however, fall into[6] the following three groups according to the basic ideas expressed. Nursing means, (1) "to **nourish**," "to cherish," "to protect," "to support"; it means "to sustain," "to **conserve** energy," "to keep in good health," and "to

impulse /ˈɪmpʌls/ n. 冲动

nourish /ˈnʌrɪʃ/ v. 滋养

conserve /kənˈsɜːv/ v. 保存

avoid injury"; (2) it means "to train," "to cultivate," "to educate," and "to supply with whatever promotes growth, development, or progress"; (3) "to give **curative** care and treatment to the sick and **infirm**."

curative /ˈkjʊərətɪv/ adj. 有疗效的
infirm /ɪnˈfɜːm/ adj. 衰弱的

6. Because nurse, like physicians, have in the past been more concerned with curative than with preventive medicine, many persons think of nurses only in connection with the care of the sick. They conceive of[7] nursing as being made up almost solely of manual skills used to bring about physical comfort and well-being. This is a limited conception of nursing, both in the unprofessional and the professional sense. A mother is nursing when she puts a **poultice**, which a physician has prescribed, on the chest of a sick child; but she is also "nursing" when she prevents a physical disease by feeding her baby cod-liver oil or checks later abnormalities of behavior by treating a temper **tantrum** wisely. Professional groups—nurses, physicians, social workers, nutritionists—as well as this mother, interpret their function to include not only the care of the sick but also the care of normal persons in the prevention of disease, and the care of the mind as well as the body. Since health conservation is the ultimate aim of all medical groups, and the work of many nurses consists entirely of health supervision, any definition that excludes preventive nursing is not only incomplete but misleading.

poultice /ˈpəʊltɪs/ n. 膏状药
tantrum /ˈtæntrəm/ n. 发脾气

7. Nursing may be defined as that service to the individual that helps him to attain or maintain a healthy state of mind or body; or,

where a return to health is not possible, the relief of pain and discomfort. This definition might apply to the work of all classes of nurses; but, because this text is written with the needs of a special group in mind, the terms nurse and nursing, as used **hereafter**, will refer to the professionally prepared and professionally minded nurse and the kind of service she gives. (752 words)

hereafter /ˌhɪərˈɑːftə(r)/ adv.（书面语）以下

Notes:

1. distinguish... from...: 区别，辨别
2. be confined to: 限制在
3. William Osler: 人名，加拿大医学家、教育家。威廉•奥斯勒（1849—1919年）是20世纪医学领域的大师，开创了现代医学新观念与新里程，是现代医学教育的始祖、临床医学的泰斗，尤其强调医学的人文与教养。他的作品《生活之道》是每一位从事医疗工作者必读的书。
4. cave dweller: 穴居人（史前石器时代）
5. yield to: 屈服
6. fall into: 分成
7. conceive of: 想象

While You Read

Task: Text-related Presentation

Directions: Take turns to make a 1-min presentation about the following topics. Your presentation should be based on the text but not limited to the text. You are encouraged to present in a unique and creative way.

1) Talk about the definition of nursing. (Para. 3)

2) Talk about the practice of nursing in the past. (Para. 4)

3) Talk about the different definitions of nursing in a dictionary. (Para. 5)

4) Talk about the limited conception of nursing and the definition of nursing in a broad sense. (Para. 6)

5) Give your understanding of nursing based on the text.

After You Read

Task 1: Academic English Study

Directions: Read this section carefully and try to find more examples of explicitness from Text A and Text B.

Explicitness

Academic writing is explicit in several ways.

1. It is explicit in its signposting of the organization of the ideas in the text. As a writer of academic English, it is your responsibility to make it clear to your reader how various parts of the text are related. These connections can be made explicit by the use of different signaling words.

a. If you want to tell your reader that your line of argument is going to change, make it clear.

Ex: Usually, *however*, she is satisfied to think of nursing in terms of what she has seen or heard. (Para. 1)

b. If you think that one sentence gives reasons for something in another sentence, make it explicit.

Ex: *Because* nurse, like physicians, have in the past been more concerned with curative than with preventive medicine, many persons think of nurses only in connection with the care of the sick. (Para. 6)

2. It is explicit in its acknowledgment of the sources of the ideas in the text.

If you know the source of the ideas you are presenting, acknowledge it.

Do THIS in academic writing

McGreil has shown that though Dubliners find the English more acceptable than the Northern Irish, Dubliners still seek a solution to the Northern problem within an all-Ireland state.

NOT

Although Dubliners find the English more acceptable than the Northern Irish, Dubliners still seek a solution to the Northern problem within an all-Ireland state.

Task 2: Critical Thinking

Directions: Work in groups and discuss the following questions. At the end of your

discussion, each group will assign a representative to present your opinions on this issue.
Nurses are traditionally and predominantly female; but during plagues that swept through Europe, male nurses were primary caregivers. In 2008, of the 3,063,163 licensed registered nurses in the United States only 6.6% of them were men. Men also make up only 13% of all new nursing students.
How do you like male nurses? Do you think men can qualify the nursing jobs? What advantages do you think male nurses have over their female counterparts?

Text B

Before You Read

Task 1: Vocabulary Preview

Directions: Preview the words in the table below and use them to describe the following pictures.

abscess shoulder blade lobar pneumonia dorsal binder bronchi

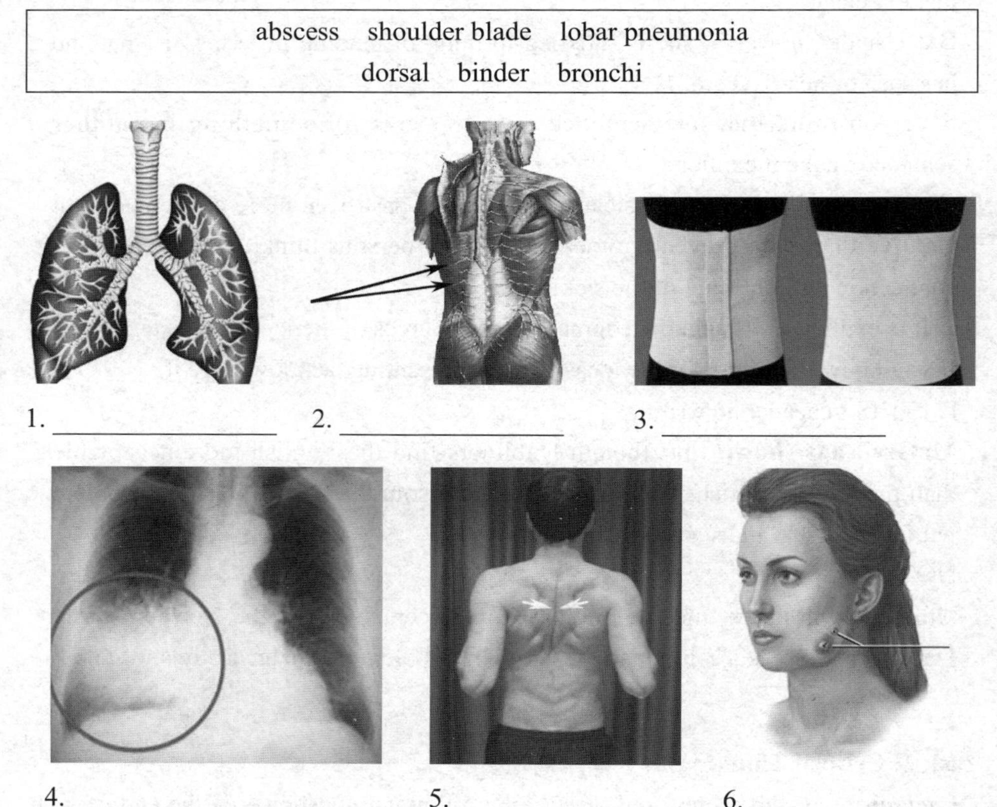

1. ________________ 2. ________________ 3. ________________

4. ________________ 5. ________________ 6. ________________

Task 2: Warming-up

Directions: Watch the video carefully and try to answer the questions below. While watching the video, please take notes in the blanks to help you follow the content.

1) What would the world be like without nurses?

2) How do nurses help patients professionally?

Notes

Text B The Plan of Care for the Patient

Case Study

An analysis of factors influencing nursing care made the second day after admission of patient as a basis for planning nursing care.

Patient: De Santo, Mrs. Angela, age, 23 yrs; nationality, U.S.A.; parentage, Italian. Service: Medical Div. A. Date of admission: 4/21/39. Discharge:

FACTORS INFLUENCING NURSING CARE	WHAT THEY SUGGEST IN TERMS OF NURSING CARE
1. *Diagnosis* (tentative): lobar pneumonia[1]? lung pneumonia? lung **abscess**? **empyema**?	1. *General nature of nursing care suggested by the diagnosis:* Care given any acute **respiratory** disease with precautions to prevent the spread of infection by discharge from the nose and throat. If presence of abscess is established, special posture will be used to favor **drainage**.

abscess /ˈæbses/ n. 脓肿

empyema /ˌempaɪˈiːmə/ n. 积脓症

respiratory /ˈrespərəˌtɔːriː/ adj. 呼吸的

drainage /ˈdreɪnɪdʒ/ n. 排水

2. *Social History and Health Record:*

(1) Family history: Grew up in an apartment in a crowded section of — with 6 sisters and brothers; father a laborer. Parents affectionate, active, emotional. The patient worked in factory from age 14 until a few months before baby was born. No record of mental disease, **tuberculosis**, or **syphilis** in the family.

(2) Marriage: One year to Michael De Santo, 24 yrs. of age, presser in a cleaning establishment. Mrs. De Santo earned $30 to $40 weekly at piece work, husband $20 to $25. They have an apartment for which they pay $35 a month. Wife resented pregnancy because it cut down income; wanted abortion. Is glad now she didn't have it; devoted to baby. Child is now with grandparents. Husband attentive and considerate on visits.

(3) Health history: Diseases of childhood, no serious illnesses; happy nature; weight has remained constant as adult (118

2. *Care must be* ***modified*** *by patient's past experience, social and economic status:*

(1) Limited economic resources suggest that patient may worry about cost of hospital care. Social service worker has been notified; has interviewed husband. Limited social and educational background makes an explanation of hospital customs and all treatment in simple terms especially important. Put patient in ward with other Italians if possible.

(2) Try to learn whether patient is worried about care given child by grandparents. If she is, suggest ways to the family of reassuring her. Encourage her to talk about the baby to comfort her for the enforced separation from her family. Later, in cooperation with social service department, investigate home to see whether conditions are suitable for **convalescence** and whether satisfactory arrangements can be made for care of child.

(3) Since Mrs. De Santo is not accustomed to[2] illness and to hospitals, especial care may be needed to prevent fear and

tuberculosis /tʊˌbɜːkjəˈləʊsɪs/ n. 肺结核

syphilis /ˈsɪfɪlɪs/ n. 梅毒

modify /ˈmɒdɪfaɪ/ v. 修改

convalescence /ˌkɒnvəˈlesns/ n. 恢复期

lbs.) except during pregnancy. Birth of child only hospital experience. "Eats everything"; drinks wine, no hard liquor; does not smoke; good appetite; tendency to **constipation**. Takes very little exercise. Appears well nourished, normal physical development.

3. *History of present illness:*
Symptoms of cold with cough, chilliness, fever, and weakness 5 days after return from maternity hospital. Visiting nurse on postpartum follow-up visit urged patient to go to bed and call doctor; this she did after second day. Patient unwilling to leave baby to care of grandmother, but was frightened by severe pain under right shoulder blade[4] that attacked her suddenly 3 days ago, and agreed to come to hospital. On admission, said she was afraid she had tuberculosis.

anxiety. She should be helped to overcome constipation through an understanding of the importance of regularity in **evacuation**, proper diet, and exercise. Measures used during illness should be designed to help establish a regular time for **defecation**.

3. *History of present illness may influence nursing care and preventive measures to be taken later:*
History of illness shows that Mrs. De Santo is very much attached to[3] her child, and this may be used to influence her later to cooperate with medical advisers, so that she can make a rapid recovery. The fact that patient is known to the local visiting nurse association means that there is one source from which information about her living conditions may be secured and that nursing supervision during convalescence is very likely available through this agency. Reassurance about the nature of her illness must be secured from the physicians if she continues to be anxious.

constipation /ˌkɒnstɪˈpeɪʃn/ n. 便秘

evacuation /ɪˌvækjʊˈeɪʃn/ n. 排泄

defecation /ˌdefəˈkeɪʃən/ n. 排便

4. *Present signs and symptoms:*	4. *Nursing care designed largely to relieve symptoms of*[5] *illness:*	
(1) Intense pain in right chest increased by deep respirations.	(1) Patient will be most comfortable lying on right side that will splint the affected lung tissue and allow freedom of movement on unaffected side. Change to **dorsal recumbent** position every 4 hours to stimulate circulation and relieve muscle strain. Support with pillows. Discourage talking; provide paper handkerchiefs and paper **sputum** cup for discharge from cough.	dorsal /ˈdɔːsl/ adj. 背部的 recumbent /rɪˈkʌmbənt/ adj. 斜倚的 sputum /ˈspjuːtəm/ n. 痰
(2) Violent episodes of coughing, with small amounts of breathing with particularly limited **excursion** in right chest. Respirations around 30 per minute.	(2) In counting respiration, place hand lightly beside left chest wall and count movements.	excursion /iksˈkəːʃən/ n. 短程旅行
(3) Temperature ranging between 38.8℃ and 39.5℃. (dropped from 40.5℃. on admission). (4) Skin pale, hot, dry; complains of sensation of chilliness much of the time.	(3 and 4) Hot-water bottle at feet will be comforting. Covering should be light and warm. As temperature **fluctuate**s, there is likely to be excessive **perspiration** and care must be taken to provide dry clothing as need arises. Important to get patient to drink large quantities of water, and high calorie diet if temperature elevation continues. Make record of intake and output of fluids.	fluctuate /ˈflʌktʃʊeɪt/ v. 波动 perspiration /ˌpɜːspəˈreɪʃn/ n. 汗水

(5) Pulse ranging between 120-130 per minute (dropped from 142 on admission). Systolic **arterial** pressure of 120, diastolic pressure 80.	(5) To lessen tax on heart, limit motor activity and emotional excitement if possible, although the increase in the pulse rate and the blood-pressure recordings indicate a fairly satisfactory reaction of the circulatory system to the **toxemia**.	arterial /ɑːˈtɪərɪəl/ adj. 动脉的 toxemia /tɒksˈiːmɪə/ n. 毒血症
(6) **Intermittent** nausea, no appetite; abdomen slightly distended.	(6) Do not force foods that are distasteful. (Ginger ale[6] is acceptable at present.) Record vomiting when it occurs, so that physician may determine need for infusion. Use cold **compresses** on forehead hot-water bottle on abdomen; **menthol** mouth wash after vomiting. Prevent unnecessary noise at bedside and avoid making the patient talk. Reduce odors to a minimum. Keep as quiet as possible.	intermittent /ˌɪntəˈmɪtənt/ adj. 间歇的 compress /kəmˈpres/ n. 敷布 menthol /ˈmenθɒl/ n. 薄荷醇
(7) Milk **exuding** from nipples; breasts slightly distended.	(7) Breasts emptied with pump twice daily or oftener if indicated. Use loose soft **binder** to keep milk from soiling gown.	exude /ɪgˈzjuːd/ v. 流出 binder /ˈbaɪndə(r)/ n.用以绑缚之物
(8) Rational but anxious. Tries to be cheerful but cries often when left alone. Looks acutely ill. Voice weak, uncertain.	(8) Give as constant nursing care and supervision as possible. Very careful explanation of all treatments. An assured, quiet, and cheerful manner on the part of the nurse may help to give Mrs. De Santo more confidence	

5. *Laboratory findings:*

(1) Blood

Hemoglobin 75 percent.

Red blood cells 3,880,000 per cm.

White blood cells 18,300 with marked increase in **polymorphonuclear** cells.

(2) Urine

No sugar, **albumin**, casts, or other abnormal **constituents**.

(3) X-ray report (not yet received).

6. *Treatment prescribed by physician:*

Date: 4-21-39.

(1) Diet-pneumonia fluids.

(2) Right side strapped.

(3) Ice-bag to right chest.

(4)Pump breasts as need is indicated.

(5) **Codeine sulphate** 0.03 gm. every 4 hours if necessary to relieve pain.

(6) Measure intake fluids and output of urine.

Date: 4-22-39.

(7) Discontinue ice-bag to chest.

(8) Apply flaxseed poultice every 4 hours to right chest.

(9) Cleansing **enema** every day if necessary.

(10) Culture of sputum.

in her chances for recovery. Conservation with her family may help to explain the cause or causes of her extreme anxiety.

5. *Laboratory findings, like diagnosis, important leads in nursing care:*

(1) Encourage patient to eat foods in prescribed diet that are high in iron content.

6. *Nursing care built around prescribed medical treatment:*

(1) Feedings scheduled about 8-10-12-3-5-8. Try out different fluids to discover which the patient likes and tolerates when nauseated.

(2) Observe skin for irritation from adhesive.

(3) Bandage ice-bags to rubber covered pillow and allow patient to lie against them.

(5) Try to relieve pain by posture and physical agents as prescribed before giving codeine, which is possibly causing nausea. Administer codeine before rest periods in the day and at night in order to get maximum benefit from the drug. Group treatments so that there will be periods in the day when patient need not be disturbed.

hemoglobin /ˌhiːməʊˈgləʊbɪn/ n. 血红蛋白

polymorphonuclear /pɒlɪmɔːfəˈnjuːkljə/ adj. 多形核的

albumin /ælˈbjuːmɪn/ n. 白蛋白

constituent /kənˈstɪtjuənt/ n. 成分

codeine /ˈkəʊdiːn/ n. 可待因

sulphate /ˈsʌlfeɪt/ n. 硫酸盐

(11) Differential blood count.

(8) Poultice should extend over **posterior** and side of right chest wall (not over breasts). Hold in place with chest binder with shoulder straps, so that patient's movements are not restricted. Binder should not be tight enough to restrict respiration.

posterior /pɒ'stɪəriə(r)/ adj. 背后的

(9) Offer bedpan after breakfast and if patient is unable to have a defecation give enema at this time to help her to establish the habit of regular defecation. Enema should also be given before bedding is changed to avoid soiling linen. Give **enema** with patient on right side in a comfortable position with legs drawn up. If effort seems to exhaust patient, report to physicians who may prefer to have a colonic irrigation[7] given.

enema /'enəmə/ n. 灌肠剂

(10) In collecting sputum, see that specimen is raised from the **bronchi** by coughing.

bronchi /'brɒŋkaɪ/ n. 细支气管

Notes:

1. lobar pneumonia: 大叶性肺炎，又名肺炎球菌肺炎，是由肺炎双球菌等细菌感染引起的呈大叶性分布的肺部急性炎症。常见诱因有受凉、劳累或淋雨等。主要病理改变为肺泡的渗出性炎症和实变。临床症状有突然寒战、高热、咳嗽、胸痛、咳铁锈色痰。血白细胞计数增高；典型的X线表现为肺段、叶实变。病程短，及时应用青霉素等抗生素治疗可获痊愈。
2. be accustomed to: 习惯于……

3. be attached to: 喜爱
4. shoulder blade: 肩胛骨，肩胛
5. relieve... of...: 减轻
6. ginger ale: 姜汁汽水
7. colonic irrigation: 结肠灌洗

While You Read

Task 1: Reading Skills Practice

Directions: Read text B carefully and try to identify the tone words in this article. Find in the corresponding paragraphs for detailed information about the methods used. (see ***Skills Bank***) Please underline the words that can reflect the author's specific tone (except the neutral tone).

Tone	Examples
optimistic	...information about her living conditions may be secured and that nursing supervision during convalescence is very likely available through this agency.
sympathetic	Limited social and educational background makes an explanation of hospital customs and all treatment in simple terms especially important.
neutral	Measures used during illness should be designed to help establish a regular time for defecation.

Task 2: Text-related Presentation

Directions:Take turns to make a 1-min presentation about the following topics.

Your presentation should be based on the text but not limited to the text. You are encouraged to present in a unique and creative way.
1) Tell us the factors influencing nursing care based on the text.
2) List the different types of personal information that has been taken into account.
3) List the present signs and symptoms of the patient.
4) What are the important leads in nursing care?

After You Read

Task 1: Oral Presenting

Directions: Try to rephrase or explain the following sentences without using the boldfaced words or phrases. (This is going to be integrated into the communicative interaction in the classroom. The task can be done orally in the classroom.)
1. Since Mrs. De Santo is not **accustomed to** illness and to hospitals, especial care may be needed to prevent fear and anxiety.
2. As temperature **fluctuates**, there is likely to be **excessive** perspiration and **care** must be **taken** to provide dry clothing as need **arises**.
3. Important to get patient to drink **large quantities of** water, and high calorie diet if **temperature elevation** continues.
4. An assured, quiet, and cheerful manner **on the part of** the nurse may help to give Mrs. De Santo more confidence in her **chances for recovery**.
5. Group treatments so that there will be periods in the day when patient need not **be disturbed**.

Task 2: Critical Thinking

Directions: Work in groups and discuss the following question. At the end of your discussion, each group will make a list of your key points in a table and select a reporter to present your opinions. The group members should take turns to report and take notes in this semester.
Based on this case study, what qualifications should a good nurse have?

After-class Tasks

Task 1: Word Chunks

Directions: Complete the following word chunks taken from Text A and Text B according to their Chinese equivalents and make a sentence with each word chunk.

1. the sick and ________ 病人和体弱者
2. ________ medicine 预防医学
3. ________ of behavior 异常行为
4. the ________ of pain and discomfort 减轻痛苦和不适
5. acute ________ disease 急性呼吸道疾病
6. ________ hospital 产科医院
7. postpartum ________ visit 产后随访
8. ________ blood circulation 促进血液循环
9. relieve muscle ________ 缓解肌肉拉伤
10. ________ and output of fluids 液体的摄入量和排出量
11. ________ rate 脉搏率
12. the ________ recording 血压的记录
13. ________ diet high in iron content 富含铁元素的处方食品
14. abnormal ________ 不正常的成分
15. ________ poultice to right chest 把药膏敷在右胸
16. ________ patients' movement 限制病人的活动
17. establish the habit of regular ________ 形成规律的排便习惯
18. ________ of sputum 痰菌培养
19. ________ blood count 血细胞分类计数
20. colonic ________ 结肠灌洗

Task 2: Translation

Directions: Translate sentence 1 to 3 into Chinese and pay close attention to the translation of words in bold. Then translate sentence 4 to 6 into English using the words in the bracket.

1. Nursing was born of the desire to protect and cherish the weak, and any expression of this desire is nursing **in the broadest sense**.

____

____

2. Nursing may be **defined as** that service to the individual that helps him to **attain** or **maintain** a healthy state of mind or body; or, where a return to health is not possible, **the relief of** pain and discomfort.

____

____

3. An analysis of factors influencing nursing care made the second day after admission of patient **as a basis for** planning nursing care.

____

____

4. 他们认为护理工作基本上只由操作技能构成，并且这些操作技能为病人带来

身体上的舒适和健康。(conceive of)

5. 因为在过去人们更多地认为护士与疾病治疗医学有关，而非预防医学，所以许多人仅仅把护士与照顾病人联系在一起。(be concerned with; in connection with)

6. 她的病史显示她对孩子的感情很深，所以这一点可以用来促进她与医学顾问的配合关系，希望她能够迅速恢复健康。(be attached to)

Task 3: Listening & Speaking

Directions: Watch the video and finish the guided note-taking before making an oral summary of what have been learnt from the video.

Word Bank

stereotype / 'stɪrɪətaɪp/ n. 老套	exclusively /ex'clusivelɪ/ adv. 专门地；排外地
disparity /dɪ'spærətɪ/ n. 不等	acquire/ ə'kwaɪə/ v. 获得

Ⅰ. Stereotype of Nurses

Ⅱ. Changing Nursing Situation

Ⅲ. Advantages of Male Nurses

Ⅳ. Future Prospects

Task 4: Research

Directions: When people hear you're a nurse practitioner, the next words out of their mouth might be, "Oh, is that under a doctor?" Do some research into the differences between a doctor and a nurse practitioner, and then brainstorm the following aspects in groups before you develop your discussions into an oral presentation for the next class. You can present in the form of an interview, short play or simply a lecture. Make sure each member of the group will present his or her part on the stage.

1) educational background
2) personality
3) care-giving style
4) salary
5) expectations from patients
6) career prospects

Resources

Here are the websites where you can find the useful information for your research.
http://rndegrees.net/difference-between-doctor-and-nurse-practitioner.php
http://medicalcareercenter.org/care-of-a-nurse-practitioner-vs-doctor-care/
http://www.neactionforhealthykids.org/nurse-practitioner-vs-doctor-which-is-the-best-choice-for-your-family/

Task 5: Writing

Directions: In January 1974, 12 May was chosen to be the Nurses' Day. Why do you think it is necessary to set aside a day to honor nurses? What are the roles of nurses? How do they change the world? Please write an essay titled "*A World without Nurses*".

Task 6: Vocabulary Log

Directions: Please finish the vocabulary log(Please find the log at the end of the book)by looking up the dictionary and write down the words or expressions you have learnt in this unit by following the examples already listed in the log. And then write down the translation for each vocabulary item and if possible, its variants, synonym, antonym and the frequent collocations.

Task 7: Reading Log

Directions: After learning the whole unit and conducting the research, you have known more about nursing from different perspectives. You can go to the library or surf on the internet for more knowledge about it. You can take down the key information according to the sample chart. (Please find the chart at the end of the book) Also you are allowed to complete the chart on a computer or tablet so that this section is expandable if you want to write more than the space on a paper form might allow. And then send it to your teacher by emails. The reading log can serve as an informal way to keep track of your reading progress.

Game

Unit 1

Directions: Divide the class into 8 groups. Each group will choose 1 card randomly from the 8 cards. When they get the card, they are going to find the word(s) from the text and figure out what it is about and the life lessons related to it. Then they are going to work together to tell a story and also the life lessons related to the word(s). Each member in the group will take turns to make up a story based on the text. Then all the other groups listen carefully and try to take notes and fill in the table below.

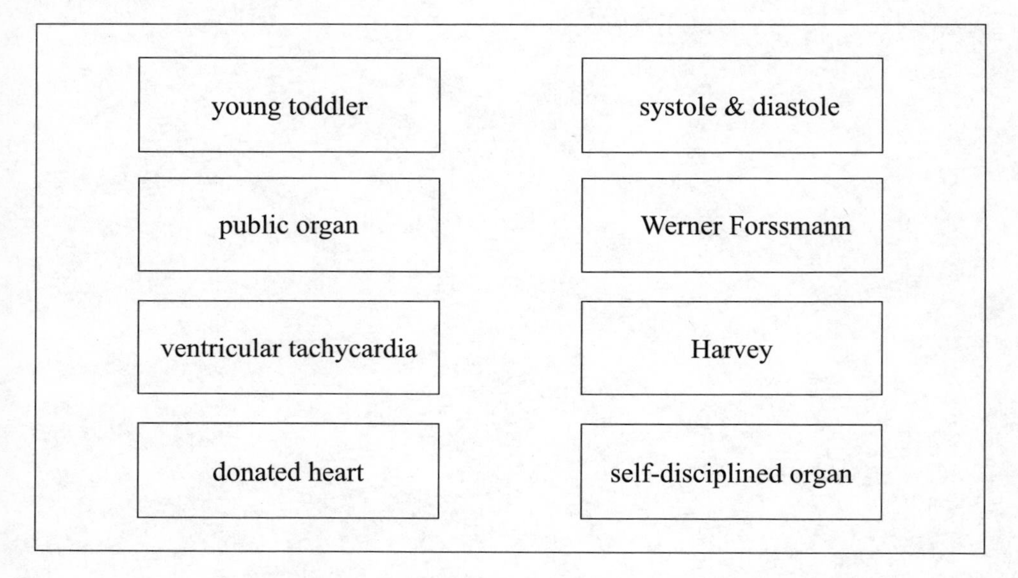

Table 1 Life Lessons from Cardiac Anatomy and Physiology

Anatomical Facts	Physiological Facts	Life Lessons

Game

Unit 2

Game 1.

Directions: Divide the class into two groups. They will compete by drawing two pictures to demonstrate the processes of John B. Gurdon's 1962 experiment (Para.5) and Shinya Nakayama's groundbreaking experiment (Para.10) half a century later respectively. The teacher acts as the judge to decide which group is the legitimate winner.

Game 2

Directions: Divide the class into two groups. They will compete by putting the steps of John B. Gurdon's 1962 experiment (Para.5) and Shinya Nakayama's groundbreaking experiment (Para.10) in correct order. The group that finishes the first wins.

Group A

1. The modified egg cell developed into a normal tadpole.
2. Gurdon replaced it with a nucleus taken from a mature cell from a tadpole.
3. Subsequent experiments involving transferal of cell nuclei have resulted in the cloning of several different mammals.
4. Gurdon destroyed the nucleus in a frog's egg.

Group B

1. Stem cells developed into all the different cell types in a mouse.
2. Shinya Yamanaka inserted genes into fibroblast cells from mouse skin.
3. Shinya Yamanaka dubbed these cells induced pluripotent stem cells (iPS cells).
4. the fibroblasts were reprogrammed and became pluripotent stem cells.

Game

Unit 3

Divide the class into several groups. Each group should get on line to find an issue regarding the art of medicine and then write the title of it on a piece of paper. A randomly selected group should explain the issue by providing detailed information. After that, the whole class can have a guess of the issue mentioned.

issue 1:	issue 7:
issue 2:	issue 8:
issue 3:	issue 9:
issue 4:	issue 10:
issue 5:	issue 11:
issue 6:	issue 12:

Game

Unit 4

The class will be divided into two sides, and each side will be further divided into several groups with 4 or 5 students in each group. Based on the information provided in Text B, one side will collect details about how doctors treat real patients at bedside and the other will collect details about how doctors treat iPatients. Then each group will find a correspondent group from the other side to perform a role-play game based on the details they have collected.

Traditional Patients	iPatient

Game

Unit 5

Directions: While learning text B, the key point is about Lister's great intellectual breakthrough. Divide the class into pairs, A and B, and give each student the appropriate section of the worksheet. Tell the students not to show each other their texts. Ask the students to read their text and write the questions they need to ask partner to complete the gap. Then, working in pairs, students take it in turns to ask and answer the questions to complete their texts. When they have finished, ask them to retell Lister's great intellectual breakthrough.

Lister's great intellectual breakthrough

A

Lister's great intellectual breakthrough came when, on the advice of Thomas Anderson, a Glasgow professor of chemistry, he read Pasteur's papers, *Recherches sur la putrefaction*,and postulated that ______________________________.
Having heard of ________ being used to disinfect sewage, he applied __________ as an antiseptic on surgical wounds. Having observed the marked difference in ____,
he postulated that infection came from exposure to the air in compound fractures without the protection of the skin. He began his antiseptic method with compound fracture wounds because ______________________________________.
The results of this new method of treating wounds were ________,and it then did not "seem right to withhold it longer from the profession generally." His work was initially published in 2 papers in the *Lancet*;______________________________

....

B

Lister's great intellectual breakthrough came when, on the advice of Thomas Anderson, a Glasgow professor of chemistry, he ____________________________,
and postulated that the same process causing fermentation was involved with wound sepsis. Having heard of creosote being used to______________ , he applied carbolic acid compounds as ____________________________. Having observed the marked difference in morbidity and mortality between simple and compound fractures, he postulated that ______________________________________.
He began his ____ because the

standard treatment of amputation was always available should his method fail. were soon apparent,and it then did not “seem right to withhold it longer from the profession generally.” ____; the first in March 1867, the second in July of the same year.

Game

Unit 6

Directions:

Divide the class into several groups. Each group will get the cards with the key words to form main ideas for the 7 paragraphs from Text B. They are required to work together to summarize using the words from the cards. The group who can finish the summary with the most words will be the winner.

1980	MASH	feasibility
1990	NASA	sense of touch
rationale	minimally invasive surgery	information system
market force	shortened recovery period	3D scanner image
"servant" tools	unaccomdating place	benefit
cost	learning curve	mishap
remote place	tight place	location

Game

Unit 7

Directions: Divide the class into several groups. Each group can get the cards to describe a person's feelings and emotions. Ask students to read Text B carefully and try to divide the words from the cards into 3 groups to describe the author's feelings before, during and after the surgery.

panic	alone	light-headed	My heart sank.	anxious
My chest was rising.		traumatized	suffocating	drowsy
I have no sensation of air moving in or out.		tachycardiac		painful
profuse sweating	relieved	distressed	rise in blood pressure	
My tongue was stuck to the roof of my mouth.				

Before the surgery	During the surgery	After the surgery

Game

Unit 8

Directions: Divide the class into pairs and give each pair section A of the worksheet. Ask them to use section A as clues to read through Text B. After 10 minutes, give each pair a jumbled set of cards cut up as indicated from section B of the worksheet. Ask the students to try to match the cards according to the text. Check the answers with the whole class and ask them to give a brief summary of the whole text using the information on the worksheet.

A	B
In a post-war era	Thalidomide was marketed to a world hooked on tranquilizers and sleeping pills
By 1960	Thalidomide was marketed in 46 countries, with sales nearly matching those of aspirin.
Around 1960	Australian obstetrician Dr. William McBride started recommending thalidomide to his pregnant patients to alleviate morning sickness setting a worldwide trend.
In 1961	McBride began to associate thalidomide with severe birth defects in the babies he delivered.
by March of 1962	Thalidomide was banned in most countries where it was previously sold
In July of 1962	President John F. Kennedy and the American press began praising FDA inspector Frances Kelsey, who prevented the drug's approval within the United States
in 1962	Passing the Kefauver-Harris Drug Amendments Act, legislators tightened restrictions surrounding the surveillance and approval process for drugs to be sold in the U.S.,
Now	Drug approval can take between eight and twelve years, involving animal testing and tightly regulated human clinical trials.

Game

Unit 9

Directions: Divide the class into groups of three to five students and give each group a set of cards. Allow students to memorize all these key words in this unit for 3 minutes or as you see fit. Pick up one student as the group leader who will hide one card each time and display the rest word cards on the desk. The other group members will see the cards carefully, find out the missing word card and tell the meaning of the word or phrase on the missing card. The student who has found the most words out will win the game.

acupuncture	TCM	herbal medicine	five-phase theory
yin-yang theory	acupoint	channels and collaterals	visceral manifestation
shadow boxing	insomnia	menopause	hormone
meditation	Confucian	ailment	illuminate
discern	complexion	gynecologist	regimen

Game

Unit 10

Directions: Divide the class into several groups. Each group can get two cards which contain two different parts of a sentence. Ask students to read Text B carefully and try to match the incomplete sentences from Card A: 1-14 with the other part from Card B: a-n. Then put the complete sentences into the five categories.

Card A	Card B
1. Get reassurance from the physicians	a. on abdomen
2. Provide paper handkerchiefs and paper sputum cup	b. in simple terms
3. Hospital customs and treatments should be explained	c. about the cost of hospital care
4. Use the patient's attachment to her son	d. before rest periods
5. Social service worker should talk with the husband	e. if the patient's anxiety continues
6. Put the patient with other Italians	f. from the local visiting nurse association
7. Obtain information about her living condition	g. before bedding is changed
8. Provide dry clothing	h. for discharge from cough
9. Encourage the patient to talk	i. from adhesive
10. Administer codeine	j. to promote her cooperation with medical advisers
11. Observe skin for irritation	k. that are high in iron content
12. Use hot-water bottle	l. about her baby
13. Advise the patient to eat foods in prescribed diet	m. if possible
14. Give enema	n. when the patient's temperature fluctuates

Care must be modified by patient's past experience, social and economic status.	
History of present illness may influence nursing care and preventive measures to be taken later.	
Nursing care designed largely to relieve symptoms of illness.	
Laboratory findings, like diagnosis, important leads in nursing care.	
Nursing care built around prescribed medical treatment.	

Vocabulary Log

Unit 1

Vocabulary Item	Chinese	Variants	Synonyms	Collocations
restless adj.	烦躁不安	n. restlessness v. rest	calm, relaxed, peaceful	the restlessness of youth get restless on sth
alternate vi. & adj.	交替	n. alternation adj. alternating adv. alternately		alternate between A and B alternate sth and/with sth
adapt vi.	适应	n. adaptation adj.adaptable	adjust,conform	quickly/easily/readily adapt to
reckless adj.	激进的			
mortality n.	死亡率			
oblivious adj.	不闻不问			
precipitate vt.	促成			
collapse vi.	崩溃			
sustain vt.	维持			
transcend vt.	超越			

Vocabulary Log

Unit 2

Vocabulary Item	Chinese	Variants	Synonyms	Collocations
contraction n.	收缩	v. contract		contraction of blood vessels
transplant v.	移植	n. transplantation		organ transplantation
culture v.	培育			culture tissue culture cells
reverse v.	反转			
convert v.	转变			
induce v.	引导			
manipulate v.	控制			
doctrine n.	学说			
hypothesis n.	假设			
hierarchy n.	等级制度			

Vocabulary Log

Unit 3

Vocabulary Item	Chinese	Variants	Synonyms	Collocations
incorporate v.	包含； 把……合并	n. incorporation adj. incorporative	combine	incorporate with
distinguished adj.	著名的；卓著的	v. distinguish	famous	distinguished guest
aggregate v., adj.	集合；聚集；合计	n. aggregation adj. aggregational	combine combined	aggregate supply aggregate performance
toxicity n.	毒性			
morbidity n.	发病率			
inpatient n.	住院病人			
empathic adj.	移情作用的			
debunk v.	揭穿			
mortality n.	死亡率			
simultaneously adv.	同时地			

Vocabulary Log

Unit 4

Vocabulary Item	Chinese	Variants	Synonyms	Collocations
trivial adj.	琐碎的，无价值的	triviality	unimportant	trivial details
corroborate v.	证实，支持	corroboration	verify	corroborate the story
methodically adv.	有系统地	method	systematically	perform methodically
abnormality n.	异常			
inadvertently adv.	由疏忽造成的			
distend v.	膨胀			
expedient adj.	方便的			
malignancy n.	恶性肿瘤			
specificity n.	特殊性			
pivotal adj.	关键的			

Vocabulary Log

Unit 5

Vocabulary Item	Chinese	Variants	Synonyms	Collocations
supersede v.	代替	ascend v. ascending adj.	replace, supplant	be superseded by...
endeavor v.	努力	endeavor n.	struggle strive	endeavor to do sth
ascent n.	升高	ascend v. ascending adj.	rise, progression	ascent to...
conversely adv.	相反地			
contagious adj.	传染的			
contamination n.	污染，感染			
sterile adj.	消毒的			
render v.	使成为； 给予			
constitute v.	组成，构成			

Vocabulary Log

Unit 6

Vocabulary Item	Chinese	Variants	Synonyms	Collocations
eliminate v.	消除	elimination n. eliminator n.	remove, dismiss, expel	eliminate sex barrier
latent adj.	潜在的	latency n.	potential	latent infection latent talent
appealing adj.	有吸引力的	appeal n.	attractive, inviting	appealing look enormously/ extremely appealing
compelling adj.	有说服力的			
inaccessible adj.	不可接近的			
unaccommodating adj.	不随和的			
advent n.	到来			
invoke v.	激发			
visionary adj.	有远见的			
inadvertently adv.	不经意地			

Vocabulary Log

Unit 7

Vocabulary Item	Chinese	Variants	Synonyms	Collocations
reversible adj.	可逆转的	reverse v. reversion n. reversal n.		reversible coat reversible kidney failure
invasive adj.	入侵性的	invade v. invasion n. invader n.		minimally invasive surgery
devastating adj.	毁灭性的	devastate v. devastation n. devastator n.	wreck destroy ruin	devastating explosion / fire / news having a devastating effect on
reassure v.	安慰			
traumatize v.	使受伤			
administer v.	给药			
numb v.	使麻木			
anesthesia n.	麻醉			
complication n.	并发症			
paralyze v.	使……瘫痪			

Vocabulary Log

Unit 8

Vocabulary Item	Chinese	Variants	Synonyms	Collocations
therapeutic adj.	治疗的	therapy n. therapist n.	curative healing alterative remedial sanative	therapeutic drug therapeutic effect therapeutic diet
prevalent adj.	发病率高的	prevalence n.	morbidity incidence	The condition is more prevalent in women than men.
alleviate v.	减轻，缓和	alleviation n.	ease sooth diminish relieve moderate	alleviate the pain
chronic adj.	慢性的			
dispense v.	分配，配药			
compound n.	化合物			
pharmacological adj.	药理学的			
sensitivity n.	敏感			
allergy n.	过敏			

Vocabulary Log

Unit 9

Vocabulary Item	Chinese	Variants	Synonyms	Collocations
discern v.	识别；领悟	discernment n. discerning adj. discernible adj.	distinguish	discernible difference
irritable adj.	急躁的；易怒的	irritate v. irritatability n.	easily annoyed	an irritable gesture
lubricate v.	润滑，使……润滑	lubrication n. lubricative adj. lubricant n.		lubricate all moving parts with grease
illuminate v.	阐明，说明			
manifestation n.	表示，显示			
formula n.	配方			
complexion n.	肤色；面色			
hormone n.	激素，荷尔蒙			
insomnia n.	失眠症，失眠			
encompass v.	包含；包围；环绕			

Vocabulary Log

Unit 10

Vocabulary Item	Chinese	Variants	Synonyms	Collocations
characterize vt.	描绘……的特征	characteristic adj & n character n.	typical, representative	be characterized by ... characterize ... as...
confine vt.	限制	confinement n. confined adj.	restrict	be confined to...
cultivate vt.	培养	cultivation n. cultivator n. cultivated adj.	foster, nurse	cultivate talents cultivate character
impulse n.	冲动			
nourish vt.	养育			
conserve vt.	保存			
conceive vi.	设想			
modify vt.	修改			
attach vt.	使依附			
fluctuate v.	波动			

Reading Log

Name: Student ID:

Date published:	Title of article:	Title of periodical:	Section:
Date accessed:	Author(s):	URL:	

Significant Points and Comments:

Something I learned:

Questions I have:

The Muddiest Points

Study Group ______		Group Members ( )		Unit ______
Items	Difficult Sentences	Viewpoints you disagree with	Your understanding of these points	Questions
Text A				
Text B				

Text-related Presentation Form

Student Name		Student ID	
Topic			

Outline

Difficulties